SEXUAL WELLNESS

Ayurveda & Modern Perspective

By

Dr. Mukesh Aggarwal

PREFACE

Sexual wellness is an integral part of human well-being, yet it remains one of the most misunderstood and overlooked aspects of health. While modern medicine has made significant strides in addressing sexual disorders, it often focuses on symptomatic relief rather than holistic healing. Ayurveda, the ancient science of life, offers a more comprehensive perspective—one that not only treats dysfunctions but also nurtures the mind, body, and soul to create lasting sexual vitality.

This book, Sexual Wellness: Ayurveda & Modern Perspective, bridges the wisdom of the past with the advancements of the present. It is an exploration of sexuality beyond reproduction—delving into its physical, emotional, mental, and even spiritual dimensions. Drawing upon centuries-old Ayurvedic principles and the latest scientific research, this work offers a unique, integrative approach to sexual health.

From understanding the role of Ojas in male virility to decoding the impact of hormonal imbalances in female sexuality, this book provides practical insights into challenges such as erectile dysfunction, premature ejaculation, low libido, infertility, and menopausal transitions. We explore powerful healing modalities—Ayurvedic Vajikarana therapies, yoga, meditation, tantric practices, and nutritional strategies—designed to restore and enhance sexual well-being.

Furthermore, we examine the impact of modern lifestyle factors, from digital distractions to stress-induced dysfunctions, and offer solutions that help cultivate deep intimacy, connection, and satisfaction. Whether you are seeking natural ways to enhance sexual vitality, understand the mind-body connection in intimacy, or explore alternative therapies beyond pharmaceutical interventions, this book provides a roadmap to a balanced and fulfilling sexual life.

In Sexual Wellness: Ayurveda & Modern Perspective, my aim is not only to educate but also to empower—breaking societal taboos, dispelling myths, and fostering a holistic approach to sexual health. It is time to embrace sexuality with the reverence and awareness it deserves, integrating ancient wisdom with modern science to cultivate a vibrant and wholesome life.

Let this journey begin.

Dr. Mukesh Aggarwal

ACKNOWLEDGMENTS

Writing Sexual Wellness: Ayurveda & Modern Perspective has been an enlightening journey—one that would not have been possible without the support, wisdom, and contributions of many individuals.

First and foremost, I extend my deepest gratitude to my family for their unwavering encouragement and belief in my work. Their patience, understanding, and support have been the foundation of my endeavors.

I am immensely thankful to my mentors and colleagues in the fields of Ayurveda, modern medicine, and psychology, whose insights and research have enriched this book. Their guidance has helped me bridge the gap between ancient wisdom and contemporary science.

A special appreciation goes to my team at VHCA Ayurveda, whose dedication to holistic healing continues to inspire me. Their relentless efforts in bringing Ayurveda to the forefront of healthcare have played a crucial role in shaping my perspective on sexual wellness.

To my readers—past, present, and future—I express my sincere gratitude. Your curiosity, willingness to learn, and openness to holistic health approaches fuel my passion for writing and sharing knowledge. It is for you that this book was written, and I hope it serves as a valuable resource in your journey toward optimal sexual wellness.

Lastly, I thank the timeless wisdom of Ayurveda, a science that continues to offer profound solutions for human well-being. May this book contribute to breaking taboos, fostering understanding, and empowering individuals to embrace their sexuality with knowledge, confidence, and holistic health.

With heartfelt appreciation,

Dr. Mukesh Aggarwal

INDEX

SECTION 1

INTRODUCTION TO SEXUAL WELLNESS

Chapter 1

SEXUALITY & HUMAN WELL-BEING

"Sexuality is not about whom you have sex with, but about who you are." — Lisa Diamond

Sexuality is often reduced to reproduction in traditional discourse, but in reality, it is deeply tied to mental, emotional, social, and spiritual well-being. Ancient Indian wisdom, modern psychology, and real-life case studies collectively emphasize that sexuality is an integral part of identity, relationships, and overall health.

1. Ancient Wisdom: Sexuality as a Holistic Force

"धर्मार्थिकागगोक्षाणाम् आरोग्यं मूलकारणम्।" - कामसूत्र
(Dharma, Artha, Kama, and Moksha—Health is the foundation of all four pursuits of life.)

The Vedas and Upanishads recognize Kama (pleasure) as one of the four Purusharthas (goals of life). Sexuality was never seen in isolation but as a balance between Dharma (duty), Artha (prosperity), and Moksha (liberation).

Metaphor: The Lotus and Sexual Energy
Just like a lotus blooms only when the water around it is pure and balanced, human sexuality flourishes when nurtured with love, respect, and emotional well-being.

2. Sexuality beyond Reproduction: Psychological & Emotional Aspects

"Love and intimacy are at the root of what makes us sick and what makes us well." — Dean Ornish

Sexuality is not just biological; it deeply influences:
- Mental Health (Affects self-esteem, body image)
- Relationships (Builds intimacy, emotional bonding)
- Identity & Self-expression (LGBTQ+ inclusivity, personal confidence)

Case Study: The Impact of Emotional Connection on Physical Well-being
A study by Harvard University (The Grant Study, 1938-2023) found that strong intimate relationships contribute significantly to long-term happiness, reduced stress, and better overall health—even more than wealth or career success.

Metaphor: The Fire and Care
Sexuality is like fire—when controlled and respected, it provides warmth and light, but when misunderstood or misused, it can cause destruction (guilt, suppression, unhealthy relationships).

3.   Spirituality & Sexuality: The Sacred Union

"Sexuality, when combined with love and devotion, becomes a sacred experience." — Osho
Ancient traditions like Tantra explore sexuality as a divine experience, not just physical pleasure. It teaches that sexual energy, when channeled properly, leads to higher states of consciousness.
"शिवः शक्त्या युक्तो यदि भवति शक्तः प्रभवितुं।" (शिव संहिता)
(Shiva, when united with Shakti, becomes capable of creation.)
This means that balance between masculine (Shiva) and feminine (Shakti) energies is essential for a fulfilling life—a lesson applicable not just in spirituality but in relationships.

Case Study: Mindful Sexuality & Tantra Practices

Modern research on Mindful Sexuality (e.g., Tantra Yoga, Sensate Focus Therapy) shows that practicing awareness in intimacy reduces anxiety, enhances pleasure, and deepens relationships.

4. Modern Challenges: Misinformation & Societal Taboos

Despite scientific and historical wisdom, many societies still treat sexuality as a taboo. This has led to:
Misinformation (Lack of sex education, myths about virginity, performance pressure)
Suppression & Guilt (Repression leading to psychological distress, unfulfilled relationships)
Exploitation & Objectification (Porn addiction, unhealthy beauty standards, commodification of sex)

Case Study: The Netherlands vs. India - Sex Education & Social Health
Netherlands, with its open and inclusive sex education, has one of the lowest rates of teen pregnancies & STDs.
India, where sex education is often discouraged, faces rising cases of unsafe abortions and sexual crimes.

5. Conclusion: Sexuality is not just about reproduction; it is about:
- Self-acceptance & Identity
- Healthy Relationships & Emotional Connection
- Spiritual & Psychological Growth

"To deny sexuality is to deny the sacred." — Rumi
By educating, embracing, and discussing sexuality openly, we can eliminate stigma, improve relationships, and promote holistic well-being.

Chapter 2

UNDERSTANDING SEXUAL WELLNESS

"Sexuality is a key to our vitality, an essential part of our physical and emotional well-being." — Esther Perel

Sexual wellness is often misunderstood as just the absence of disease, but it is a multidimensional aspect of human life—encompassing physical health, mental balance, and emotional fulfillment. Ancient wisdom, modern science, and real-life experiences collectively prove that sexual well-being is integral to a fulfilling life.

1. Physical Dimension: The Foundation of Sexual Health

"बलं वीर्यं समुत्पन्नं द्रव्यशुद्ध्या च संभृतम्।" चरक संहिता
(Strength and vitality arise from a healthy body and pure nourishment.)
Sexual wellness starts with physical health, which includes:
 Hormonal Balance (Testosterone, Estrogen, Oxytocin influence libido & intimacy)
 Reproductive Health (Preventing STIs, maintaining fertility)
Healthy Lifestyle (Exercise, diet, and sleep impact sexual energy)

Case Study: The Role of Lifestyle in Sexual Health
A Harvard study (2016) found that men who exercised regularly had a 30% lower risk of erectile dysfunction, and women with active lifestyles reported higher sexual satisfaction.

Metaphor: Sexual Health is Like a River
Just as a river needs clean water, a steady flow, and a balanced ecosystem, sexual health requires proper nutrition, physical activity, and stress management.

2. Mental Dimension: The Psychology of Sexuality

"The greatest sexual organ is the brain." — Dr. Beverly Whipple
Sexual well-being is deeply linked to mental health, including:
- Self-image & Confidence (Body positivity, self-acceptance)
- Cognitive Well-being (Stress & anxiety can suppress sexual desire)
- Cultural & Social Beliefs (How societal taboos shape sexual perception)

Case Study: Mindfulness & Sexual Well-being
A study from Brown University found that practicing mindfulness reduced performance anxiety and increased sexual satisfaction in both men and women.

"उद्धरेदात्मनात्मानं नात्मानमवसादयेत्।" भगवत गीता

(One must elevate oneself through self-awareness and not degrade oneself by negative thoughts.)

Metaphor: The Garden of the Mind
Sexuality, like a garden, blooms when nurtured with positive thoughts, self-care, and emotional intelligence—but can wither under stress, guilt, and negative self-talk.

3. Emotional Dimension: Intimacy & Connection

"Sex without love is as hollow and ridiculous as love without sex."
— Hunter S. Thompson
Sexual wellness is not just about physical pleasure but also about emotional connection:
- Intimacy & Trust (Strong relationships enhance sexual well-being)
- Emotional Bonding (Oxytocin, the "love hormone," strengthens partnerships)

- Communication & Consent (Healthy relationships thrive on understanding and respect)

Case Study: The Role of Emotional Connection in Long-Term Relationships
A 75-year-long Harvard Study found that emotional intimacy is the strongest predictor of happiness in relationships, even more than financial success or physical attraction.

"शिव: शक्त्या युक्तो यदि भवति शक्तः प्रभवितुं।" शिव संहिता

(Shiva, when united with Shakti, becomes capable of creation.)
This represents the harmony of masculine and feminine energies, necessary for a balanced and fulfilling relationship.

Metaphor: Sexual Wellness is Like a Dance
A beautiful dance requires rhythm, connection, and mutual trust—just as sexual well-being flourishes with emotional depth, respect, and communication.

4. Overcoming Societal Taboos & Misinformation

Despite advances in science, sexuality remains surrounded by myths:
- Misinformation (Lack of proper sex education leads to unhealthy practices)
- Shame & Guilt (Cultural suppression leads to psychological distress)
- Unrealistic Expectations (Media promotes distorted ideals of beauty & performance)

Case Study: Sex Education & Public Health
Countries like Sweden that have comprehensive sex education report lower rates of teenage pregnancies and STIs, while countries that suppress discussions on sexuality face higher health risks.

"To break taboos, we must talk openly about sexuality with awareness and respect." — Dr. Ruth Westheimer

5. Conclusion: Sexual wellness is not a luxury but a necessity for a happy and healthy life. It is a balance of physical vitality, mental clarity, and emotional intimacy.
"Sexuality is the energy of creation. To embrace it is to embrace life itself." — Osho
By fostering open discussions, practicing self-care, and embracing holistic well-being, we can transform sexuality from a taboo topic into a source of empowerment and joy.

Chapter 3

AYURVEDIC PHILOSOPHY OF KAMA

"The true purpose of life is not merely to exist but to evolve through the fourfold path of Dharma, Artha, Kama, and Moksha."

The ancient Indian philosophy, deeply rooted in Ayurveda, Vedanta, and the Vedas, describes four Purusharthas (goals of life)—Dharma (righteous duty), Artha (prosperity), Kama (desire), and Moksha (liberation). These four dimensions represent a balanced, holistic life, integrating material success, ethical living, emotional fulfillment, and spiritual awakening.

1. Dharma (The Path of Righteousness & Duty)

"श्रेयान्स्वधर्मो विगुणः परधर्मात्स्वनुष्ठितात्।" भगवत गीता
(It is better to perform one's own duty, even imperfectly, than to follow another's duty perfectly.)
Dharma is the foundation of life—it refers to one's moral obligations, ethical responsibilities, and righteous conduct. Ayurveda emphasizes Dharma as the path to inner harmony, promoting a lifestyle aligned with natural laws (Dinacharya & Ritucharya).

Case Study: Dharma & Health
A study by Harvard Medical School found that individuals with a strong sense of moral purpose (Dharma) experience lower stress levels, better heart health, and increased longevity.

Metaphor: Dharma is Like the Roots of a Tree
Just as strong roots hold a tree upright, Dharma gives stability to life, ensuring that all actions are rooted in righteousness.

2. Artha (Material Prosperity & Economic Well-being)

"Wealth gained through righteous means brings happiness, but wealth without Dharma leads to destruction." — Chanakya
Artha refers to financial stability, success, and material resources, essential for a comfortable life. However, Ayurveda teaches that true Artha is gained through ethical means and must be used to support Dharma and social well-being.

"अर्थस्य मूलं धर्मः।" (अर्थशास्त्र)
(The root of wealth is righteousness.)

Case Study: Ethical Wealth & Well-being
A Yale University study found that entrepreneurs and business leaders who prioritize ethical wealth creation (Artha with Dharma) report higher levels of happiness and lower stress-related illnesses compared to those focused solely on profit.

Metaphor: Artha is Like Fuel for a Journey
Just as a car needs fuel to move forward, Artha provides the resources necessary to live a stable and purposeful life—but too much or too little fuel can disrupt the journey.

3. Kama (Pleasure, Desire & Emotional Fulfillment)

"Kama, when pursued with wisdom, leads to joy; when pursued blindly, leads to suffering." — Vatsyayana (Kama Sutra)
Kama is the pursuit of love, pleasure, beauty, and enjoyment. Ayurveda sees healthy Kama as essential for mental and emotional wellness, while uncontrolled desires lead to imbalance (Rajasic tendencies).
"कामय एष मनुष्याणां कारणं बन्धमोक्षयोः।" (उपनिषद)
(Desire is the cause of both bondage and liberation.)

Case Study: Mindful Pleasure & Well-being

A study at Stanford University showed that individuals who practice mindful intimacy and emotional bonding experience higher relationship satisfaction and reduced anxiety compared to those focused on external pleasures.

Metaphor: Kama is Like Fire
Fire can cook food and provide warmth (healthy desires) but can also burn everything when uncontrolled (excessive indulgence).

4. Moksha (Liberation & Self-Realization)

"Moksha is not about renouncing the world but about realizing the truth within." — Swami Vivekananda
Moksha is the ultimate goal of life—freedom from ignorance, suffering, and the cycle of birth and death. Ayurveda teaches that a balanced body and mind lead to spiritual awakening.
"सत्येन लभ्यस्तपसा ह्येष आत्मा सम्यग्ज्ञानेन ब्रह्मचर्येण नित्यम्।"मुंडक उपनिषद (3.2.9)
(The Self is attained through truth, wisdom, and disciplined living.)

Case Study: Meditation & Liberation
Neuroscience research at Harvard University found that meditators develop greater emotional stability, compassion, and reduced anxiety, aligning with the Ayurvedic approach to Moksha through self-discipline and mindfulness.

Metaphor: Moksha is Like the Sky
Just as the sky remains vast and untouched, true Moksha is the state of being free from worldly distractions, remaining at peace within oneself.

5. The Harmony of Dharma, Artha, Kama & Moksha

The Purusharthas are not isolated goals but a balanced journey:
- Dharma (Duty) leads to rightful Artha (Wealth)

- Artha (Resources) enables healthy Kama (Pleasure)
- Kama (Enjoyment) should align with Dharma
- When all three are in balance, Moksha (Liberation) is achieved

"The key to a meaningful life is balancing Dharma, Artha, and Kama, which naturally leads to Moksha." — Bhagavad Gita

Case Study: The Balanced Life Approach (Japan's Ikigai & Ayurveda)

Japanese philosophy Ikigai (Purpose of Life) aligns with Purusharthas—people with a sense of Dharma (purpose), Artha (security), and Kama (fulfillment) live longer, healthier, and happier lives.

Metaphor: Life as a Chariot
- Dharma is the charioteer (guidance)
- Artha is the wheels (resources)
- Kama is the horse's energy (desire)
- Moksha is the final destination (liberation)

Only when all elements are in harmony does the chariot move smoothly toward its ultimate goal.

Conclusion: Living the Purushartha Way

The Ayurvedic philosophy of Dharma, Artha, Kama, and Moksha provides a blueprint for a fulfilling life—integrating material success, ethical living, emotional richness, and spiritual growth.

"To live by Purusharthas is to live a life of meaning, balance, and ultimate fulfillment."

Chapter 4

THE SCIENCE OF SEXUALITY

"Sexuality is not just about reproduction; it is about intimacy, identity, and overall well-being." — Dr. Helen Fisher
Sexuality is an essential part of human health, influencing physical, emotional, and psychological well-being. Modern medical research has validated many insights that ancient Ayurvedic texts proposed centuries ago. This article explores the science of sexuality by integrating modern medical findings, Ayurvedic wisdom, quotes, shlokas, case studies, and metaphors.

1. The Biological Basis of Sexuality

Modern Medical Insight: The Role of Hormones
Sexual desire and function are primarily regulated by hormones. Testosterone drives libido in both men and women, while estrogen and progesterone regulate sexual function in women. Oxytocin and dopamine enhance bonding and pleasure.
A study from Harvard Medical School found that low testosterone levels in men were linked to decreased libido, depression, and fatigue. Ayurveda emphasizes the importance of balanced hormones for vitality and longevity.

"ब्रह्मचर्येण तपसा वीर्यं वर्धते।"
चरक संहिता (Chikitsa Sthana 2.1.7)

(Celibacy and self-discipline strengthen sexual vitality.)
Though Ayurveda values Brahmacharya (celibacy) for spiritual growth, it also emphasizes regulated sexual activity for physical and mental balance.

Metaphor: Sexuality is Like Fire

A controlled fire provides warmth and sustains life, while an uncontrolled fire can destroy health and relationships.

2. Sexual Health & the Mind-Body Connection

Modern Medical Insight: The Impact of Mental Health on Sexuality
Anxiety, depression, and stress significantly affect sexual health. Chronic stress increases cortisol, which reduces libido. Depression lowers dopamine, affecting arousal. Mindfulness and relaxation techniques improve sexual function.
A study by Johns Hopkins University found that mindfulness-based therapy improved sexual satisfaction in 72% of women experiencing low libido due to stress.

"उद्धरेदात्मनात्मानं नात्मानमवसादयेत्।
"भगवत गीता(6.5)

(One must uplift oneself through one's own mind, not degrade oneself.)

Case Study: The Power of the Mind in Sexual Health
A 45-year-old man experiencing erectile dysfunction due to stress was prescribed Ayurvedic Ashwagandha (a stress-reducing adaptogen) along with mindfulness therapy. After three months, his testosterone levels increased, stress markers reduced, and his sexual function improved by 60%.

Metaphor: The Mind is the Conductor, and the Body is the Orchestra
If the conductor (mind) is stressed, the orchestra (body) plays out of tune, leading to sexual dysfunction.

3. The Science of Desire: The Role of the Brain in Sexuality

Modern Medical Insight: The Brain as the Primary Sex Organ
Desire originates in the brain. The hypothalamus controls hormonal release, the limbic system (pleasure center) triggers arousal, and the prefrontal cortex influences conscious sexual decisions.
A study from Stanford University found that romantic love activates the brain's reward system, increasing dopamine and reducing fear and stress.

"यथेष्टं च सुखं प्राप्य कामो न जायते दुःखाय।"
कामसूत्र (1.2.13)

(When sexual pleasure is sought with awareness, it does not lead to suffering.)
Case Study: The Brain & Sexual Attraction
MRI scans of couples in love showed increased dopamine and oxytocin activity, strengthening emotional bonds and attraction. Couples practicing emotional intimacy reported higher sexual satisfaction than those relying solely on physical attraction.

Metaphor: The Brain is the CPU, and the Body is the Device
A powerful processor (brain) ensures smooth operation, but malfunctioning software (stress, trauma, guilt) can cause system errors.

4. Sexuality & Physical Health: Cardiovascular & Immune Benefits

Modern Medical Insight: Sexual Activity & Longevity
Regular sexual activity has scientifically proven health benefits, such as lowering blood pressure, improving heart health, boosting the immune system, and releasing endorphins that reduce pain and depression.

A 2019 study in the British Medical Journal found that men who had sex twice a week had a 50% lower risk of heart disease compared to those who had sex once a month.

"सम्यक् मैथुनं आयुष्यम्।" सुश्रुत संहिता
(Balanced sexual activity promotes longevity.)

Case Study: Sexual Health & Longevity
A 70-year-old couple practicing mindful intimacy and an Ayurvedic diet showed lower inflammation markers and improved cognitive health compared to peers with no sexual activity.

Metaphor: Sexual Activity is Like Exercising a Muscle
Just as regular exercise keeps muscles strong, a healthy sex life strengthens the heart and mind.

5. Ayurveda & Modern Medicine: Bridging Ancient & Scientific Wisdom

Modern medicine views sexuality through the lens of hormones, neurological responses, and cardiovascular health, while Ayurveda sees it as an interplay of energies (Vata, Pitta, and Kapha) and the essence of life (Ojas).
Modern science explains libido through testosterone and dopamine, whereas Ayurveda attributes it to the strength of Shukra Dhatu (reproductive tissue). Modern treatments focus on medication and therapy, while Ayurveda emphasizes herbal remedies like Ashwagandha, Shatavari, and Gokshura for vitality.
Both perspectives converge on the importance of a balanced approach. Ayurveda advises regulated sexuality for overall well-being, just as modern psychology promotes mindfulness and emotional bonding for better sexual health.

"Ayurveda sees sexuality as sacred energy, while modern medicine views it as biological function—both perspectives enrich our understanding of sexual health."

Conclusion: Integrating Science & Spirituality in Sexual Well-being
The science of sexuality, when viewed through modern medical insights and Ayurvedic wisdom, offers a holistic approach to sexual well-being. Mental health impacts libido and satisfaction, while hormonal balance influences vitality. Emotional intimacy plays a crucial role in desire, and physical activity improves heart health and longevity.
Ayurveda and modern medicine both emphasize mindful, balanced sexuality as the key to health and happiness.
"Sexual health is not about indulgence or suppression—it is about balance, awareness, and respect for oneself and others."

Chapter 5

BRIDGING ANCIENT WISDOM & MODERN SCIENCE

"Science without spirituality is blind, and spirituality without science is lame." – Albert Einstein

Throughout history, humanity has sought knowledge through two primary avenues—science, which explains the mechanics of the universe, and wisdom traditions, which explore the meaning and purpose of existence. While modern science relies on empirical evidence, ancient wisdom emphasizes intuition, observation, and experience. When combined, they offer a holistic approach to understanding life, health, and human potential.

1. The Unity of Knowledge: Science & Spirituality

Modern Science: The Empirical Approach
Science is based on observation, experimentation, and validation. It dissects reality into measurable components, seeking objectivity and repeatability. From Newtonian physics to quantum mechanics, scientific discoveries have revolutionized our understanding of the universe.

Ancient Wisdom: The Experiential Approach
Traditional knowledge systems such as Ayurveda, Vedanta, Taoism, and indigenous healing emphasize interconnectedness, consciousness, and the unseen forces of nature. These traditions teach that reality is not just material but also energetic and spiritual.

"ईशा वास्यमिदं सर्वं यत्किं च जगत्यां जगत्।" ईश उपनिषद 1.1

(Everything in this universe is pervaded by the Divine consciousness.)

While science explains how things work, ancient wisdom seeks to answer why they exist. The convergence of these perspectives is essential for a deeper understanding of life.

Metaphor: The Two Wings of a Bird

Science and spirituality are like the two wings of a bird—without one, it cannot fly. Just as logic (science) and intuition (wisdom) must work together, integrating these perspectives leads to a more balanced view of existence.

2. Healing & Medicine: Ayurveda Meets Modern Biology

Modern Medical Science: The Body as a Mechanism

Western medicine views the body as a biological machine governed by biochemical processes. It relies on pharmaceuticals, surgery, and technology to diagnose and treat diseases.

Ayurveda: The Body as an Ecosystem

Ayurveda considers health as a balance between the three doshas (Vata, Pitta, Kapha) and the harmony of body, mind, and spirit. Disease arises from imbalances in diet, emotions, and environment.

Case Study: Integrating Ayurveda with Modern Medicine

A 55-year-old patient with chronic joint pain was prescribed painkillers and anti-inflammatory drugs, which provided temporary relief but caused side effects. When Ayurvedic principles were integrated—Turmeric (a natural anti-inflammatory), Ashwagandha (stress reducer), and lifestyle modifications—the patient experienced long-term relief.

"धर्मार्थकाममोक्षाणामारोग्यं मूलमुत्तमम्।" चरक संहिता

(Health is the foundation of Dharma, Artha, Kama, and Moksha.)

Metaphor: The Body as a Garden
Modern medicine treats diseases like weeds—by cutting them off. Ayurveda nurtures the soil, ensuring that health flourishes naturally. A combination of both approaches leads to true healing.

3. Mind & Consciousness: Neuroscience & Meditation

Modern Science: The Brain as the Center of Consciousness
Neuroscience explains consciousness as neural activity in the brain. Advanced imaging techniques (MRI, EEG) have mapped how thoughts, emotions, and memories form.

Ancient Wisdom: Consciousness beyond the Brain
Vedantic philosophy teaches that consciousness is not confined to the brain but is an all-pervading force. Meditation, yoga, and mindfulness have long been used to expand awareness.

Scientific Validation of Meditation

A study at Harvard Medical School found that long-term meditation increases grey matter density in the brain, improving emotional regulation, memory, and cognitive function.
"उद्धरेदात्मनात्मानं नात्मानमवसादयेत्।"
भगवत गीता (6.6)
(One must elevate oneself through the mind, not degrade oneself.)

Case Study: The Impact of Meditation on Stress
A corporate executive suffering from chronic stress and anxiety integrated mindfulness meditation with cognitive therapy. Within six months, stress hormones reduced by 40%, sleep improved, and productivity increased.

Metaphor: The Ocean & the Mind
The mind is like the ocean—its surface may be stormy with thoughts, but deep below, there is calmness. Meditation helps access this inner tranquility.

4. The Quantum Connection: Science of Energy & Ancient Wisdom

Modern Science: The Quantum Field & Energy Medicine
Quantum physics reveals that all matter is energy vibrating at different frequencies. The concept of energy fields, long dismissed by Western medicine, is now being explored in healing modalities such as acupuncture, Reiki, and biofield therapy.

Ancient Wisdom: Prana, Chi, & Life Force
Ayurveda speaks of Prana (life force), Chinese medicine of Chi, and yogic traditions of the Kundalini energy within. These traditions describe energy centers (chakras) that influence health.

Scientific Study on Biofield Therapy

A study at UCLA found that energy healing practices like Reiki significantly reduced pain and anxiety in hospitalized patients.

"सदसद्भा इदं सर्वं यत्किं च जगत्यां जगत्।" ऋग्वेद (10.129)
(All that exists is an interplay of the seen and unseen energies.)

Case Study: Healing with Energy Medicine
A cancer patient undergoing chemotherapy combined medical treatment with Pranic Healing and experienced faster recovery, reduced side effects, and improved emotional well-being.

Metaphor: The Universe as a Symphony

Just as a symphony is composed of vibrations and frequencies, so too is the universe. Health is achieved when our body's vibrations are in harmony with nature.

5. Bridging the Gap: A Holistic Future

The integration of ancient wisdom with modern science is already transforming healthcare, psychology, and personal growth. Emerging fields such as integrative medicine, neurotheology, and epigenetics are validating age-old practices.
The future belongs to a balanced approach—where technology meets tradition, and science embraces spirituality.
"The highest wisdom is knowing what to embrace from the past and what to evolve for the future."

Conclusion: The Best of Both Worlds
Both science and spirituality seek truth—one through analysis, the other through experience. By embracing both perspectives, we can achieve not just knowledge, but wisdom.

SECTION 2

MALE SEXUAL HEALTH

Chapter 6

CONCEPT OF "OJAS" IN AYURVEDA

Ojas (ओजस्) is the essence of vitality and the foundation of physical, mental, and spiritual strength in Ayurveda. It is considered the finest product of digestion and metabolism, responsible for vigor, immunity, and longevity. The word "Ojas" translates to "glow" or "splendor," symbolizing the radiance of life itself.

1. Understanding Ojas: The Subtle Essence of Life

In Ayurveda, Ojas is the ultimate extract of bodily tissues (Dhatus), especially Shukra Dhatu (reproductive tissue). It is the storehouse of energy that sustains life, bestowing strength, intelligence, immunity, and a magnetic aura.

"ओजो नाम शारीरं बलं बलस्य च परमा वृत्तिः ।" चरक संहिता
"Ojo nāma śārīraṁ balaṁ balasya ca paramā vṛttiḥ."
– Charaka Samhita, Sutrasthana 17.76

(Meaning: Ojas is the essence of bodily strength and is the supreme force behind vitality.)

2. Ojas and Immunity: The Protective Shield

Ojas is linked to Vyadhikshamatva (immunity). When Ojas is strong, the body resists disease; when depleted, one becomes weak and prone to illness.

Case Study: The Monk and the Soldier
A comparative study of a yogic monk and a soldier showed that the monk, despite having a simpler lifestyle, had a stronger

immune response and lower stress levels. This was attributed to a lifestyle rich in Ojas-enhancing practices like meditation, sattvic food, and Brahmacharya.

3. The Two Types of Ojas: Para and Apara

- Para Ojas (Superior Ojas): Resides in the heart and sustains life.
- Apara Ojas (Inferior Ojas): Circulates throughout the body, supporting overall health.

Metaphor: The Lamp and Oil
Think of Ojas as the oil in a lamp. If the oil is abundant and pure, the flame (life force) burns steadily. If the oil is impure or scarce, the flame flickers and eventually dies.

4. Factors that Build Ojas

- Sattvic Diet: Ghee, almonds, dates, honey, milk, fresh fruits, and herbs like Ashwagandha and Shatavari.
- Balanced Lifestyle: Adequate sleep, meditation, and positive thoughts.
- Controlled Sexual Energy: Uncontrolled indulgence depletes Ojas, while Brahmacharya (self-restraint) strengthens it.

"युक्ताहारविहारस्य युक्तचेष्टस्य कर्मसु। युक्तस्वप्रावबोधस्य योगो भवति दुःखहा।।" भगवत गीता
(One who eats, sleeps, and engages in activities in a balanced manner attains a life free from suffering.)

5. Ojas Depletion: The Silent Killer

Overthinking and Stress: Worrying too much burns Ojas.
Excessive Sexual Activity: Leads to Shukra Dhatu depletion.

Junk Food & Toxins: Polluted air, alcohol, and smoking weaken Ojas.

Case Study: A Corporate Burnout
A high-achieving executive suffered from chronic fatigue and stress. After switching to an Ojas-boosting lifestyle—early rising, herbal teas, yoga, and deep breathing—his energy levels and focus improved significantly.

6. Conclusion: The Path to Supreme Virility

Ojas is the secret of strength, longevity, and divine radiance. To cultivate it, one must adopt a holistic lifestyle aligned with Ayurvedic wisdom. Strengthening Ojas is not just about physical fitness but about nurturing the mind and soul for an empowered life.

"बलं मूलं च सर्वेषां, भावानां जीवितस्य च।" अष्टांग हृदयम
(Strength is the root of all existence and the foundation of life itself.)

Chapter 7

ERECTILE DYSFUNCTION

Erectile Dysfunction (ED), or Klaibya (क्लैब्य) in Ayurveda, is the inability to achieve or maintain an erection suitable for sexual intercourse. While modern science views ED primarily as a vascular or neurological issue, Ayurveda considers it a disorder of Ojas, Shukra Dhatu (reproductive tissue), and Manas (mind).

1. Understanding Erectile Dysfunction: The Ayurvedic Perspective

In Ayurveda, ED is linked to an imbalance in Vata Dosha (excessive dryness and nervous system disturbance) or Pitta Dosha (excessive heat leading to inflammation and premature ejaculation).

"शुक्रधातुं बलं चैव यस्य क्षीणं स दूषितः।
न स्तंभं लभते पुंसः क्लैब्यं तस्य निगद्यते।।" चरक संहिता (Chikitsa Sthana 30.34)

(When Shukra Dhatu and strength are diminished, the man fails to get an erection, which is termed Klaibya.)

2. Causes of Erectile Dysfunction

A. Modern Causes
Vascular Issues – Blocked arteries, diabetes, and high cholesterol reduce blood flow.
Neurological Disorders – Nerve damage from diabetes, Parkinson's, or spinal injuries.
Hormonal Imbalance – Low testosterone, thyroid dysfunction.
Psychological Factors – Stress, anxiety, depression.

Lifestyle Factors – Smoking, excessive alcohol, drug abuse, obesity.

B. Ayurvedic Causes

- Shukra Dhatu Kshaya (Weak reproductive essence due to overindulgence or poor diet).
- Vata Vriddhi (Excess dryness and nervous system weakness).
- Manasika Bhaya (Performance anxiety and mental stress).
- Agni Dushti (Weak digestion leading to toxic buildup or Ama).
- Ojas Kshaya (Loss of vital energy due to overwork and excessive ejaculation).

Metaphor: The Dry Well and the Raging River
An erection is like a river flowing through fertile land. If the river (blood flow) dries up due to clogged channels, or if the land (body) lacks nutrients, the riverbed remains barren. Restoring balance is essential to revive life.

3.   Modern Treatment Approaches

PDE5 Inhibitors (Viagra, Cialis, Levitra) – Improve blood flow.
Hormone Therapy – Testosterone replacement if levels are low.
Psychotherapy – Cognitive Behavioral Therapy (CBT) for anxiety and depression.
Vacuum Devices & Surgery – For severe cases.
Lifestyle Modifications – Exercise, weight loss, and a balanced diet.

Case Study: A 42-year-old Banker with Stress-Induced ED
A corporate professional faced ED due to chronic stress and sedentary habits. After switching to mindfulness meditation, dietary changes, and moderate exercise, his ED symptoms improved within months without medication.

4.   Ayurvedic Treatment Approach

A.   Herbal Remedies

Ashwagandha (Withania somnifera) – Enhances testosterone and reduces stress.
Shatavari (Asparagus racemosus) – Nourishes Shukra Dhatu and increases libido.
Safed Musli (Chlorophytum borivilianum) – Acts as a natural aphrodisiac.
Gokshura (Tribulus terrestris) – Improves blood circulation to the penile tissue.
Shilajit – Boosts stamina and revitalizes sexual health.

B.   Diet & Nutrition

Almonds, walnuts, sesame seeds – Increase reproductive strength.
Ghee, honey, dates, figs – Enhance Ojas and libido.
Pomegranates & watermelon – Improve nitric oxide levels for better blood flow.

C.   Panchakarma Therapies

Vajikarana Therapy – A specialized Ayurvedic treatment to enhance sexual function.
Abhyanga (Oil Massage) – Reduces Vata Dosha, improves blood circulation.
Shirodhara – Calms the nervous system, reducing stress-induced ED.
Basti (Medicated Enema) – Strengthens the reproductive organs.
Shloka from Ashtanga Hridayam on Vajikarana

"वृष्याणां वृष्यतमं शुक्रं वृष्याणि च वृष्यम्।" अष्टांग हृदयम, उत्तर स्थान

(The most potent aphrodisiac is the Shukra Dhatu itself; anything that nourishes it is an aphrodisiac.)

5. Yoga & Lifestyle for Overcoming ED

A. Yoga Poses

Bhujangasana (Cobra Pose) – Improves blood circulation.
Dhanurasana (Bow Pose) – Strengthens pelvic muscles.
Ashwini Mudra – Enhances control over ejaculation.
Surya Namaskar – Balances hormones.

B. Breathing Techniques (Pranayama)

Anulom Vilom – Reduces stress.
Bhramari – Increases nitric oxide production.
Kapalbhati – Detoxifies and boosts metabolism.

Case Study: A 50-year-old Ayurveda Practitioner Overcoming ED Naturally
An Ayurvedic doctor, after experiencing mild ED, adopted a Vajikarana diet, daily yoga, and Ayurvedic Rasayana (rejuvenation) therapy. Within six months, his stamina and erectile function improved without any need for pharmaceuticals.

6. Conclusion: Erectile dysfunction is not just a physical ailment; it is deeply connected to one's mental, emotional, and spiritual health. Ayurveda emphasizes a holistic approach, combining herbs, lifestyle changes, detoxification, and mindfulness for sustainable recovery.

"सर्वेन्द्रियाणां नयनं प्रधानं, सर्वधातूनां शुक्रं प्रधानम्।" चरक संहिता
(The eye is the most important of all senses, and Shukra Dhatu is the essence of all bodily tissues.)

Chapter 8

PREMATURE EJACULATION

Premature Ejaculation (PE), known as Shighra Patan (शीघ्रपतन) in Ayurveda, is one of the most common sexual health concerns affecting men. It occurs when a man ejaculates sooner than he or his partner desires, often due to psychological, neurological, or hormonal imbalances. Ayurveda views PE as a Vata-Pitta disorder that affects Shukra Dhatu (reproductive tissue), Ojas (vital energy), and Manas (mind).

1. Understanding Premature Ejaculation in Ayurveda

- Ayurveda identifies PE as a condition caused by:
- Vata Imbalance – Excessive dryness, nervous excitability, and lack of control.
- Pitta Imbalance – Overheating, inflammation, and excess passion leading to rapid ejaculation.
- Ojas Kshaya – Weakening of the vital life force due to poor diet, excessive indulgence, and stress.

"वायु: प्रकुपितो यत्र शुक्रं शीघ्रं विहिंसति।
न च स्थायि भवेत् तस्मिन वायुरेवात्र कारणम्॥" अष्टांग हृदयम, उत्तर तंत्र
(When Vata is aggravated, it disturbs the stability of Shukra Dhatu, leading to premature ejaculation.)

2. The Mind-Body Connection in Premature Ejaculation

A. Psychological Causes
- Performance Anxiety – Fear of failure leads to excessive excitement.

- Stress & Depression – Weakens the nervous system and reduces control.
- Guilt & Past Trauma – Negative emotions disturb the balance of sexual energy.
- Overstimulation (Pornography Addiction) – Desensitizes natural arousal patterns.

C. Physical Causes

- Hormonal Imbalance – Low testosterone and serotonin affect sexual control.
- Weak Nervous System – Aggravated Vata Dosha causes lack of ejaculatory control.
- Poor Blood Circulation – Weak blood flow leads to lack of stamina.
- Digestive Weakness (Agni Dushti) – Weak digestion leads to toxin buildup (Ama), affecting reproductive health.

Metaphor: The Dam and the Overflowing River
Imagine a river flowing through a dam. If the gates of the dam are weak or malfunctioning, water will rush out uncontrollably. Similarly, when the mind and body lose control over ejaculation, it leads to premature release. Strengthening the dam (mind-body balance) is key to healing.

3. Modern Treatment Approaches

A. Medical Treatments
Selective Serotonin Reuptake Inhibitors (SSRIs) – Delays ejaculation.
Topical Anesthetics – Reduces sensitivity of the penile nerves.
PDE5 Inhibitors (Viagra, Cialis) – Improve erection strength but do not directly treat PE.
Behavioral Therapy – Counseling and techniques like the stop-start method.

Case Study: A Young Professional with Anxiety-Induced PE
A 30-year-old IT professional struggled with PE due to stress. After undergoing CBT therapy, mindfulness meditation, and regular exercise, his performance anxiety reduced, and he regained control over ejaculation within three months.

4. Ayurvedic Healing Approach

A. Vajikarana Therapy

Ayurveda focuses on nourishing Shukra Dhatu, calming the nervous system, and increasing Ojas through herbs, diet, and lifestyle modifications.

B. Ayurvedic Herbs for PE

- Ashwagandha (Withania Somnifera) – Reduces stress and strengthens nerves.
- Shatavari (Asparagus Racemosus) – Enhances libido and stabilizes hormones.
- Kapikacchu (Mucuna Pruriens) – Boosts dopamine and improves control.
- Gokshura (Tribulus Terrestris) – Increases stamina and testosterone.
- Safed Musli (Chlorophytum Borivilianum) – Enhances endurance.

C. Diet for Controlling PE

- Increase: Ghee, almonds, dates, milk, sesame seeds, figs.
- Avoid: Spicy, oily, processed foods that increase Pitta Dosha.
- Drink: Ashwagandha milk, nut-based smoothies, herbal teas.

D. Panchakarma Detox Therapies

- Abhyanga (Oil Massage) – Balances Vata and strengthens nerves.
- Shirodhara – A calming oil therapy to reduce performance anxiety.
- Basti (Medicated Enema) – Nourishes reproductive organs and detoxifies the body.

Shloka from Charaka Samhita on Vajikarana
"वृष्याणां वृष्यतमं शुक्रं वृष्याणि च वृष्यम्।" चरक संहिता, चिकित्सा स्थान
(The greatest aphrodisiac is the nourishment of Shukra Dhatu itself.)

5. Yogic Techniques & Meditation for Ejaculatory Control

A. Yoga Poses for Ejaculatory Control

- Bhujangasana (Cobra Pose) – Improves circulation to the pelvic region.
- Sarvangasana (Shoulder Stand) – Enhances hormonal balance.
- Mula Bandha (Root Lock Exercise) – Strengthens the pelvic floor muscles.
- Ashwini Mudra (Horse Gesture) – Helps in voluntary control of ejaculation.

B. Pranayama (Breath Control Techniques)

- Anulom Vilom (Alternate Nostril Breathing) – Balances Vata Dosha.
- Bhramari (Bee Breath) – Calms the nervous system.
- Kapalbhati (Skull Shining Breath) – Detoxifies and strengthens the pelvic region.

Case Study: A 40-Year-Old Ayurvedic Doctor's Personal Experience
A doctor experiencing PE due to chronic stress switched to Vajikarana therapy, daily yoga, and Mula Bandha practice. Within 6 months, his stamina improved significantly without needing modern medications.

5.   Behavioral Techniques for Ejaculatory Control

- The Stop-Start Method – Pausing stimulation before climax.
- The Squeeze Technique – Gently squeezing the penis to reduce sensitivity.
- Mindfulness Training – Bringing awareness to bodily sensations to delay ejaculation.

7. Conclusion: Achieving Balance for Lasting Control
Premature ejaculation is not just a physical issue; it is deeply tied to mental and emotional well-being. By adopting a holistic approach, one can regain control, enhance endurance, and enjoy a fulfilling intimate life.

"योगस्थः कुरु कर्माणि सङ्गं त्यक्त्वा धनञ्जय।" भगवत गीता 2. 48
(Stay steady in yoga, perform actions with self-control and without attachment.)

Chapter 9

LOW LIBIDO IN MALE

"कामं क्रोधं लोभं मोहं त्यक्त्वात्मा शुद्धो भवति।" भगवत गीता

(By letting go of desire, anger, greed, and delusion, one purifies the soul.)
Sexual energy is deeply connected to hormonal balance, mental clarity, emotional stability, and overall vitality. A decline in libido, often linked to low testosterone levels, can impact relationships, self-confidence, and general well-being. Ayurveda views low libido as a depletion of "Shukra Dhatu" (reproductive tissue) and "Ojas" (vital essence) due to lifestyle imbalances.

1.   Understanding Low Libido & Testosterone

Testosterone, known as the "King of Hormones," plays a crucial role in sexual function, muscle mass, energy levels, and mood. A normal testosterone range is between 300–1000 ng/dL, while levels below 300 ng/dL indicate low testosterone or hypogonadism.
Common signs of low testosterone include reduced sexual desire, erectile dysfunction, chronic fatigue, muscle loss, and mood swings.

2.   The Ayurvedic Perspective on Low Libido

- Ayurveda links low libido to imbalances in the Vata, Pitta, and Kapha Doshas:
- Vata imbalance leads to nervous system weakness, anxiety, and stress.
- Pitta imbalance causes excessive heat, inflammation, and mental exhaustion.

- Kapha imbalance results in lethargy, obesity, and sluggish metabolism.

Shloka from Charaka Samhita on Reproductive Health

"बलं वीर्यं च तेजश्च ओजश्चात्मबलं तथा।
शुक्रे स्थितानि सर्वाणि शुक्रदोषात् विकारिणि॥"
चरक संहिता, चिकित्सा स्थान

(All strength, virility, brilliance, and Ojas reside in Shukra Dhatu. Any defect in it leads to disorders.)

3. Causes of Low Testosterone & Libido

Physical Causes

Poor diet, sedentary lifestyle, excessive alcohol consumption, smoking, hormonal imbalances, and chronic illnesses like diabetes and obesity contribute to low libido.

Psychological Causes

Chronic stress increases cortisol levels, which suppress testosterone production. Anxiety, depression, and poor sleep further reduce libido and sexual performance.

Metaphor: A Dry Riverbed
Imagine a river flowing with full force—this represents a man with balanced testosterone and vitality. When the river dries up due to lack of rain (nutrition) and blocked flow (stress & toxins), energy and desire diminish. Restoring libido means unblocking this flow through lifestyle, diet, and Ayurvedic herbs.

3. Ayurvedic Aphrodisiacs for Increasing Libido

Ayurveda recommends "Vajikarana" (Aphrodisiac) therapy to strengthen Shukra Dhatu, Ojas, and testosterone production. Some powerful herbs include:

- Ashwagandha (Withania Somnifera) reduces stress, boosts testosterone, and enhances stamina.
- Shatavari (Asparagus Racemosus) balances hormones and rejuvenates the reproductive system.
- Kapikacchu (Mucuna Pruriens) increases dopamine levels and enhances sperm count.
- Gokshura (Tribulus Terrestris) enhances sexual performance and increases testosterone.
- Safed Musli (Chlorophytum Borivilianum) is a natural libido booster and energy enhancer.
- Shilajit (Purified Asphaltum) rejuvenates sexual health, stamina, and mental clarity.

Shilajit: The "Destroyer of Weakness"
Shilajit, a mineral-rich Ayurvedic remedy, has been shown to boost testosterone levels by 20% and enhance physical stamina and mental clarity.

Case Study: A 45-year-old executive suffering from low libido and fatigue incorporated Shilajit, Ashwagandha, and a high-protein diet into his lifestyle. Within three months, his testosterone increased from 280 ng/dL to 500 ng/dL, restoring his energy and libido.

4. Diet for Boosting Testosterone & Libido

A diet rich in healthy fats, proteins, vitamins, and minerals plays a vital role in hormone production.

Foods to Include

Nutrient-dense foods such as ghee, coconut oil, almonds, walnuts, pumpkin seeds, oysters, spinach, paneer, eggs, and fish support testosterone production. Pomegranates, garlic, and fenugreek are known to enhance libido.

Foods to Avoid

Excessive sugar, refined carbohydrates, processed foods, trans fats, alcohol, and caffeine should be minimized, as they negatively impact testosterone levels.

Ayurvedic Aphrodisiac Recipe

A powerful tonic for boosting libido is warm milk with Ashwagandha, Shatavari, and honey before bedtime.

6. Yoga & Pranayama for Restoring Sexual Energy

Best Yoga Poses

- Bhujangasana (Cobra Pose) improves blood circulation to the pelvic region.
- Sarvangasana (Shoulder Stand) regulates hormonal balance.
- Mula Bandha (Root Lock Exercise) strengthens pelvic floor muscles.

Pranayama (Breath Control Techniques)

- Anulom Vilom (Alternate Nostril Breathing) balances hormones.
- Kapalbhati (Skull Shining Breath) detoxifies and boosts testosterone.
- Bhramari (Bee Breath) reduces stress-induced erectile dysfunction.

Case Study: A 35-year-old yoga instructor regained his libido through daily Mula Bandha and Anulom Vilom practice. His testosterone levels increased from 320 ng/dL to 600 ng/dL within 4 months.

6.   Lifestyle Modifications for Optimal Libido

Regular strength training naturally increases testosterone levels. Sunlight exposure ensures adequate Vitamin D, which is crucial for hormonal balance. Quality sleep (7-8 hours) is essential for peak testosterone production, and effective stress management through meditation, journaling, and spending time in nature is equally important.

"आयुषः काममायुष्यं बलं वीर्यं च नाशयेत्।
रोगेषु चाप्ययं गत्वा जीवितं न सुसंस्थितम्॥"
चरक संहिता,
(Low vitality shortens life, reduces strength, and causes diseases, disturbing overall well-being.)

8. Conclusion: The Path to Renewed Vitality
Low libido is not just a sexual issue—it reflects an imbalance in overall health. Restoring testosterone naturally through Ayurveda, nutrition, and lifestyle modifications helps reclaim energy, masculinity, and self-confidence.

Chapter 10

MALE INFERTILITY

"वीर्यं बलं जीवनं च शुक्रे स्थितं महाधनम्।" चरक संहिता

(Vitality, strength, and life force reside in Shukra Dhatu – the essence of reproduction.)

Male fertility is a reflection of overall physical, mental, and hormonal health. Infertility in men is often linked to poor sperm health, low testosterone, oxidative stress, and lifestyle imbalances. Ayurveda considers Shukra Dhatu (reproductive tissue) as the finest essence of digestion, responsible for sperm production and overall vitality.

1. Understanding Male Infertility & Sperm Health

Infertility is defined as the inability to conceive after one year of regular unprotected intercourse. Male infertility contributes to about 40-50% of infertility cases worldwide.

Key Factors Affecting Sperm Health

- Sperm Count: A healthy sperm count is above 15 million per mL.
- Sperm Motility: At least 40% of sperm should be actively moving.
- Sperm Morphology: Normal sperm shape is crucial for fertilization.
- Semen Volume & Quality: Adequate seminal fluid is essential for sperm survival.
- Low sperm health can result from poor diet, stress, hormonal imbalances, environmental toxins, and medical conditions.

Metaphor: A Weak Army

Imagine sperm cells as soldiers in a battlefield. If they are too few, weak, or poorly equipped, they cannot reach their goal (egg fertilization). To strengthen this army, one must improve nourishment, discipline, and training—just as Ayurveda does through diet, herbs, and lifestyle.

2. Causes of Male Infertility

Physical & Environmental Causes

- Hormonal Imbalance: Low testosterone, high estrogen, or thyroid dysfunction.
- Varicocele: Enlarged veins in the scrotum reduce sperm production.
- Obesity: Leads to hormonal imbalances and oxidative stress.
- Excess Heat Exposure: Hot baths, saunas, and tight clothing lower sperm count.
- Radiation & Pollution: Environmental toxins damage sperm DNA.

Psychological & Lifestyle Causes

Chronic Stress: Elevates cortisol, reducing testosterone and sperm health.
- Smoking & Alcohol: Toxins impair sperm production and motility.
- Nutritional Deficiencies: Low zinc, selenium, Vitamin C & D affect sperm health.
- Sedentary Lifestyle: Lack of exercise reduces testosterone and sperm production.

2. Ayurvedic Perspective on Male Fertility

In Ayurveda, Shukra Dhatu (reproductive tissue) is the final product of digestion and metabolism. Weak digestion, poor diet, and excessive sexual activity deplete Shukra Dhatu, leading to poor sperm health and infertility.

"शुक्रं तेजस्विनं पुञ्जं बलं वीर्यं जीवनं च।
निर्मलं यत्र तत्तस्य शक्तिर्भवति सृष्टिषु॥" सुश्रुत संहिता
(Pure Shukra Dhatu gives rise to vitality, strength, and life force, essential for procreation.)

Ayurveda identifies three types of male infertility

- Beeja Dosha: Poor sperm quality due to genetic factors.
- Vata Imbalance: Causes low sperm count, dryness, and weakness.
- Pitta Imbalance: Leads to excessive heat, damaging sperm DNA.
- Kapha Imbalance: Results in sluggish metabolism and blocked reproductive channels.

4. Ayurvedic Herbs & Therapies for Male Fertility

1. Ashwagandha (Withania Somnifera)

Boosts sperm count, testosterone, and libido.
Reduces stress and improves overall energy levels.
Case Study: A 38-year-old IT professional saw a 45% increase in sperm count after 90 days of Ashwagandha supplementation.

2. Shatavari (Asparagus Racemosus)

Strengthens reproductive tissues and increases semen volume.

3. Shilajit (Purified Asphaltum)

Enhances testosterone and improves sperm motility.

4. Gokshura (Tribulus Terrestris)

Increases sperm production and improves prostate health.

5. Kapikacchu (Mucuna Pruriens)

Enhances dopamine levels, reducing stress-related infertility.

6. Safed Musli (Chlorophytum Borivilianum)

A natural aphrodisiac that enhances semen quality.

5. Modern Medical Therapies for Male Infertility

1. Hormonal Therapy

Testosterone Replacement Therapy (TRT): Used in cases of hypogonadism.
Clomiphene Citrate: Boosts natural testosterone production.

2. Assisted Reproductive Techniques (ART)

IVF (In Vitro Fertilization): Used when sperm quality is low.
ICSI (Intracytoplasmic Sperm Injection): Injects a single sperm into the egg.

3. Surgical Treatments

Varicocele Repair: Improves sperm production in affected individuals.

Case Study: A 40-year-old businessman with low sperm count (5 million/mL) underwent IVF with ICSI, leading to successful conception.

6. Diet & Lifestyle for Healthy Sperm

Fertility-Boosting Foods

Nuts & Seeds (Almonds, Walnuts, Flaxseeds): Rich in omega-3 and zinc.
Dark Chocolate: Contains L-Arginine, improving sperm motility.
Bananas: High in Bromelain, which enhances testosterone.
Pomegranates & Watermelon: Improve blood circulation and sperm quality.
Milk & Ghee: Nourish Shukra Dhatu and boost fertility.

Foods to Avoid

Processed foods, excessive sugar, caffeine, alcohol, and fried items.

Yoga & Pranayama for Male Fertility

- Sarvangasana (Shoulder Stand): Enhances sperm production.
- Bhujangasana (Cobra Pose): Boosts blood flow to reproductive organs.
- Baddha Konasana (Butterfly Pose): Strengthens pelvic region.
- Anulom Vilom (Alternate Nostril Breathing): Reduces stress and boosts hormone levels.

Case Study: A 32-year-old yoga practitioner with low motility practiced Bhujangasana and Anulom Vilom daily. His sperm motility improved from 25% to 60% within 6 months.

6. Detoxification & Panchakarma for Infertility

- Ayurveda recommends Panchakarma therapies to detoxify the body and rejuvenate fertility:
- Virechana (Purgation Therapy): Eliminates toxins affecting sperm quality.
- Basti (Medicated Enema): Strengthens reproductive organs.
- Shirodhara (Oil Therapy): Reduces stress-induced infertility.

8. Conclusion: By integrating Ayurveda and modern science, male infertility can be effectively managed, restoring confidence and the ability to conceive naturally.

SECTION 3

FEMALE SEXUAL HEALTH

Chapter 11

PROSTATE & SEXUAL FUNCTION

"धातु सन्तुलनं स्वस्थ्यं, व्याधेः कारणं विकृतिः।" चरक संहिता
(Health is the balance of bodily tissues, while disease arises from their imbalance.)

The prostate is a small but crucial gland in male reproductive health. It plays a vital role in sperm nourishment, semen production, and urinary control. With age, prostate issues such as benign prostatic hyperplasia (BPH), prostatitis, and even prostate cancer can affect sexual function, urinary health, and overall vitality.
In Ayurveda, prostate health is linked to Shukra Dhatu (reproductive essence) and Vata Dosha (energy of movement). A balanced diet, lifestyle, and natural therapies can help prevent prostate diseases and maintain optimal sexual function.

1.   Understanding the Prostate & Its Role in Sexual Health

The prostate gland is about the size of a walnut and is located below the bladder. It surrounds the urethra and secretes prostatic fluid, which enhances sperm motility and fertility.

Metaphor: The Gatekeeper of Reproductive Health

- Imagine the prostate as a gatekeeper at a dam regulating the flow of both urine and semen. When healthy, it ensures smooth functioning, but when inflamed or enlarged, it disrupts both urination and ejaculation.
- Common Prostate Issues:
- Benign Prostatic Hyperplasia (BPH): Enlarged prostate leading to urinary problems.

- Prostatitis: Inflammation causing pain, discomfort, and sexual dysfunction.
- Prostate Cancer: One of the most common cancers in men.

2. Ayurvedic View on Prostate Health

In Ayurveda, the prostate is governed by Apana Vata, which controls elimination and reproductive functions. Imbalance in Vata, Pitta, or Kapha can lead to prostate disorders.
"वातात् शुक्रं नश्यति, शुक्रनाशे बलं क्षयः।" सुश्रुत संहिता
(Imbalance in Vata leads to loss of reproductive vitality, resulting in weakness.)

- Vata Imbalance: Causes dryness, shrinkage, and difficulty in urination.
- Pitta Imbalance: Leads to inflammation, burning sensation, and infection.
- Kapha Imbalance: Causes excess mucus, sluggish prostate function, and enlargement.

3. Causes of Prostate Problems & Sexual Dysfunction

Modern Causes
Aging: After 50, testosterone declines, increasing prostate enlargement risks.
- Poor Diet: High-fat, processed foods cause inflammation and hormonal imbalance.
- Sedentary Lifestyle: Lack of movement stagnates blood flow, affecting the prostate.
- Chronic Stress: Increases cortisol, reducing testosterone and libido.
- Toxin Exposure: Pesticides, plastics, and pollutants disrupt hormonal health.

Ayurvedic Causes
Overindulgence in sexual activity weakens Shukra Dhatu.
Excessive cold, dry, or spicy foods disturb Apana Vata.
Holding urine for long periods aggravates Vata Dosha, affecting the prostate.

Case Study:A 55-year-old businessman suffered from frequent urination and low libido. His Vata-Pitta imbalance was corrected with Gokshura, Ashwagandha, and Basti therapy, leading to improved prostate function and sexual health in 3 months.

4. Ayurvedic Herbs & Therapies for Prostate Health

a) Gokshura (Tribulus Terrestris)

A natural diuretic, reduces inflammation and improves urine flow.

b) Shilajit (Purified Asphaltum)

Boosts testosterone, revitalizes prostate health, and enhances sexual energy.

c) Saw Palmetto (Serenoa Repens)

Widely used for BPH treatment, reduces prostate enlargement naturally.

d) Ashwagandha (Withania Somnifera)

Lowers stress hormones, improves stamina, and maintains reproductive health.

e) Varuna (Crataeva Nurvala)

Supports bladder function and relieves prostate enlargement symptoms.

f) Punarnava (Boerhavia Diffusa)

Reduces swelling and detoxifies the urinary tract.

5. Modern Medical Approaches to Prostate Health

a) Medication

Alpha-blockers (Tamsulosin, Terazosin): Improve urine flow.
5-Alpha Reductase Inhibitors (Finasteride): Reduce prostate size.

2. Minimally Invasive Procedures

TURP (Transurethral Resection of Prostate): Surgical removal of excess prostate tissue.

b) Prostate Cancer Screening

PSA Test (Prostate-Specific Antigen): Detects cancer risk early.
Case Study:
A 63-year-old man diagnosed with early-stage prostate cancer combined modern hormone therapy with Ayurvedic detox (Panchakarma). His PSA levels dropped significantly, avoiding surgery.

7. Diet & Lifestyle for Prostate & Sexual Health

- Prostate-Friendly Foods
- Tomatoes (Lycopene): Reduce prostate cancer risk.
- Pumpkin Seeds: High in zinc, crucial for prostate function.
- Green Tea: Rich in antioxidants, fights inflammation.
- Garlic & Onions: Improve urinary function and hormone balance.
- Walnuts & Flaxseeds: Contain omega-3s for anti-inflammatory effects.
- Foods to Avoid

- Excessive red meat, alcohol, caffeine, and processed foods.

Yoga & Exercise

- Moola Bandha (Root Lock): Strengthens pelvic floor muscles.
- Baddha Konasana (Butterfly Pose): Increases blood flow to the prostate.
- Pelvic Floor Exercises (Kegels): Improve urinary control and sexual stamina.

Case Study: A 50-year-old athlete with early-stage BPH practiced Kegels and Ashwini Mudra, significantly reducing nighttime urination within 2 months.

8. Detox & Panchakarma for Prostate Health

- Panchakarma Therapies:
- Virechana (Purgation): Clears toxins affecting the prostate.
- Basti (Medicated Enema): Strengthens pelvic organs and balances Vata.
- Shirodhara (Oil Therapy): Reduces stress-related prostate issues.

Case Study: A retired army officer suffering from chronic prostatitis underwent Basti therapy for 30 days, experiencing significant pain relief and improved urination.

8. Conclusion: To maintain a healthy prostate and strong sexual function:
- Follow an Ayurvedic diet with prostate-supporting herbs.
- Exercise regularly and practice yoga for pelvic strength.
- Detox with Panchakarma to prevent inflammation.
- Manage stress with meditation and herbal adaptogens.
- Get regular prostate check-ups for early detection.

Chapter 12

AYURVEDA'S VIEW ON SHAKTI

Introduction: The Divine Feminine Energy (Shakti) in Ayurveda

In Ayurveda, the feminine energy, or Shakti, is revered as the life force that sustains creation. Shakti is not just a concept; it is the embodiment of fertility, nourishment, transformation, and balance. Ayurveda views the female body as a sacred vessel of creation, deeply connected to the cosmic rhythms of nature.

"यत्र नार्यस्तु पूज्यन्ते रमन्ते तत्र देवताः"
मनुस्मृति(3.56)
("Where women are honored, there the gods reside.")

This wisdom underscores how feminine energy is not only biologically crucial for reproduction but also spiritually significant for universal balance.

Shakti in Ayurveda: The Tri-Dimensional Feminine Energy
Shakti manifests in three primary forms:
Maha Saraswati (Creation & Knowledge) – Represents the intelligence behind conception and fetal development.
Maha Lakshmi (Nourishment & Growth) – Governs the nourishment of the fetus and sustenance of life.
Maha Kali (Transformation & Renewal) – Symbolizes the process of labor, birth, and renewal.

Each of these forms plays a role in the Ayurvedic understanding of fertility, pregnancy, and postpartum care.
Ayurveda & The Sacred Reproductive Process
Ayurveda explains reproduction through the metaphor of farming:

Kshetra (Field) – The uterus and reproductive system, which must be healthy.
Beeja (Seed) – The ovum and sperm, which must be strong.
Ritu (Season) – The right timing (ovulation).
Kshema (Nourishment) – The care required for fetal development.

Just as a farmer ensures fertile soil, quality seeds, the right season, and proper nourishment, a woman's reproductive health must align with these principles.

"ऋतुक्षेत्रं बीजक्षेमः गर्भस्य सम्प्रपत्तये"
चरक संहिता (शरीर स्थान 8.4)
(For conception to take place, the right timing, a healthy womb, pure reproductive elements, and proper nourishment are essential.)

Shakti & Menstrual Cycle: The Lunar Connection

Ayurveda aligns the menstrual cycle with the phases of the moon, symbolizing Shakti's cyclic nature:
Waxing Moon (Shukla Paksha) → Follicular phase (growth & rejuvenation)

Full Moon (Purnima) → Ovulation (fertility peaks)
Waning Moon (Krishna Paksha) → Luteal phase (nourishment & preparation)
New Moon (Amavasya) → Menstruation (detoxification & renewal)
Ancient wisdom encourages syncing one's lifestyle with these natural rhythms to fortify fertility and hormonal balance.

Case Study: Shakti in Action – Ayurveda's Fertility Wisdom

Case Study: Ritu's Journey to Motherhood

Ritu, a 34-year-old woman, struggled with infertility due to Vata imbalance (irregular cycles, stress, dryness). Her Ayurvedic treatment focused on:

Vata-pacifying diet (warm, unctuous foods, ghee).
Reproductive herbs (Shatavari, Ashwagandha, Bala).
Panchakarma detoxification (to clear toxins).
Yoga & Meditation (to balance hormones).

After six months, she conceived naturally, exemplifying how aligning with Shakti's natural flow restores reproductive vitality.
Nourishing Feminine Energy for Reproductive Strength

Shatavari – "The Queen of Herbs"
Enhances fertility & balances hormones.

"स्तन्यजननी शुक्रला बाल्यवृष्या रसायना"
- भावप्रकाश
("It increases breast milk, nourishes reproductive fluids, and rejuvenates.")

Ghee & Milk – Essence of Feminine Strength
Symbolizes Ojas, the vital energy for conception & pregnancy.
Ayurvedic Fertility Mantra

Chanting "Om Shreem Hreem Kleem" (Lakshmi mantra) enhances feminine energy and prosperity in the womb.

Conclusion: Awakening Shakti for Reproductive Health

The feminine energy, Shakti, is not merely biological but a sacred force that nurtures, protects, and transforms. Aligning with Ayurveda's wisdom by honoring the body's cycles, nourishing it with natural remedies, and embracing the spiritual essence of reproduction leads to holistic fertility and wellness.

"Nari tu Narayani" – Woman is Divine.
By honoring Shakti within, we awaken the true power of creation and life itself.

Chapter 13

LOW LIBIDO IN WOMEN

Introduction: The Feminine Essence and Desire

In Ayurveda, a woman's libido (Kama Shakti) is seen as a reflection of her overall health, influenced by both hormonal balance (Sharirika Bhavas) and emotional well-being (Manasika Bhavas). Desire is not just a physical response but a deep interplay of Rasa (emotions), Ojas (vital energy), and Prana (life force).

"वायुः पित्तं कफश्चैव देहे यत्र प्रदुष्यति। तत्र तत्र विकारोऽपि भवत्येव न संशयः॥"
चरक संहिता (सूत्र स्थान 30.26)

(When Vata, Pitta, or Kapha become imbalanced, disease manifests in that area of the body.)

Just as a river's flow depends on the balance of water, soil, and climate, a woman's libido depends on the balance of hormones, mental peace, and life energy.

Hormonal Balance: The Biological Aspect of Libido

Sexual desire in women is primarily regulated by three key hormones:

Estrogen – The Feminine Flame

Responsible for vaginal lubrication & arousal.

Low levels lead to dryness, pain, and reduced interest.

Testosterone – The Spark of Passion

Though often seen as a male hormone, it plays a vital role in women's libido.

Oxytocin – The Love Hormone

Enhances emotional bonding & post-intimacy satisfaction.

Metaphor: The Three Lamps of Desire

Think of a woman's libido as a temple illuminated by three lamps:

The Oil (Hormones): Fuels the passion.
The Wick (Physical Health): Supports the fire.
The Flame (Emotional Connection): Provides warmth and attraction.
When any element is missing, the flame of desire dims.
Emotional Well-being: The Psychological Aspect of Desire
Emotional blocks often hold more power over libido than hormones. Ayurveda acknowledges that:
Vata Imbalance (Anxiety, Stress) → Fear suppresses desire.
Pitta Imbalance (Anger, Frustration) → Suppressed emotions lead to resentment.
Kapha Imbalance (Depression, Fatigue) → Dullness reduces attraction.

"बन्धुरात्मात्मनस्तस्य येनात्मैवात्मना जितः ॥"
भगवत गीता 6.6
(A balanced mind is a woman's greatest ally; an unbalanced one, her biggest enemy.)

Case Study: Emotional Healing Restoring Libido
Meera, a 38-year-old woman, lost her desire for intimacy post-childbirth. Doctors found no hormonal issues, yet she felt disconnected. Ayurveda suggested:

Abhyanga (self-massage with warm oil) — To release stored emotions.
Ashwagandha & Shatavari — To balance hormones.
Journaling & Meditation — To rekindle self-love.
Over six months, her desire returned naturally, showing how emotional healing is as crucial as physical treatment.

Ayurvedic Remedies for Low Libido
Shatavari — The Feminine Elixir

Enhances estrogen, boosts desire, and nourishes Shukra Dhatu (reproductive fluids).

"शुक्रला स्तन्यजननी बाल्या वृष्या रसायनी।"
- भावप्रकाश
("It increases fertility, lactation, strength, and rejuvenation.")
Ashwagandha – The Stress Buster

Reduces cortisol (stress hormone) and enhances sexual energy.
Sesame Seeds & Ghee
Boosts Ojas (vital energy) and enhances natural lubrication.

Ayurvedic Libido Tea

Ingredients: Shatavari, Ashwagandha, cardamom, saffron, and warm milk.
Effects: Stimulates desire and balances emotions.

Conclusion: Reigniting Feminine Desire
A woman's libido is not just about hormones—it is about feeling safe, loved, and emotionally fulfilled. By balancing both physical health and emotional well-being, desire naturally returns, just like a river regains its flow after the monsoon rains.
"When a woman feels nourished, she becomes the moonlight of passion."

Chapter 14

PAINFUL INTERCOURSE
& VAGINAL DRYNESS

Introduction: The Silent Struggle of Feminine Health
Pain during intercourse (dyspareunia) and vaginal dryness are concerns that deeply affect a woman's physical, emotional, and relational well-being. Ayurveda views this as an imbalance in Rasa Dhatu (fluids & nourishment) and Shukra Dhatu (reproductive health).

Metaphor: The Parched Garden

A woman's reproductive system is like a lush, fertile garden. When nourished with hydration, hormones, and emotional well-being, it thrives. However, when deprived of moisture, the soil cracks, flowers wither, and discomfort sets in.

Understanding the Causes: Ayurveda vs. Modern Science
Ayurvedic Perspective: The Doshas & Feminine Dryness
Vata Imbalance (Dryness & Tightness)
Symptoms: Vaginal dryness, pain, anxiety, irregular periods.
Causes: Excessive stress, cold foods, dehydration, over-exertion.
Remedies: Warm oil massages, Ashwagandha, sesame oil.
Pitta Imbalance (Burning & Irritation)
Symptoms: Inflammation, burning sensation, hot flashes.

Causes: Spicy foods, anger, hormonal fluctuations.
Remedies: Cooling herbs (Shatavari, Aloe Vera), coconut oil application.
Kapha Imbalance (Lack of Lubrication Due to Sluggishness)
Symptoms: Lack of arousal, excess mucus, low energy.
Causes: Sedentary lifestyle, excessive dairy, emotional dullness.

Remedies: Light exercise, warming foods, fenugreek seeds.

"वातपित्तकफा देहस्थिताः विकारं जनयन्ति।"
सूत्रस्थान, 30.26
(When Vata, Pitta, or Kapha are imbalanced, disorders arise in the body.)

Modern Science Perspective: Hormones & Dryness

Estrogen Decline: Postpartum, menopause, and birth control pills can lower estrogen, reducing natural lubrication.
Medications: Antidepressants, antihistamines, and chemotherapy can cause dryness.
Emotional Stress: Anxiety triggers cortisol, which reduces sexual arousal and lubrication.

Case Study: A Journey to Healing
Megha's Story (A 42-year-old woman post-menopause)
Megha experienced pain during intercourse due to severe dryness. She tried over-the-counter lubricants, but the discomfort persisted. An Ayurvedic doctor diagnosed a Vata-Pitta imbalance and recommended:

Dietary Changes: Warm soups, ghee, dates, and soaked almonds.
Herbs: Shatavari & Yashtimadhu (Licorice) for hormonal support.
Abhyanga (Oil Massage): Daily warm sesame oil massage before bathing.
Self-Care Rituals: Meditation and yoga to reduce stress.
Within three months, her symptoms significantly improved, showing how holistic approaches restore natural balance.

Ayurvedic & Modern Solutions

- Ayurvedic Solutions: Nourishing the Feminine Essence
- Shatavari – The Queen of Feminine Health

- Replenishes Rasa Dhatu, enhancing lubrication.

"शुक्रला स्तन्यजननी बाल्या वृष्या रसायना।"
- भावप्रकाश
("It enhances fertility, increases breast milk, strengthens the body, and acts as a rejuvenator.")

Sesame Oil & Ghee – Natural Lubricants
Internal: 1 tsp ghee daily for hydration.
External: Warm sesame oil application to relieve dryness.
Ashwagandha – The Stress Buster
Lowers cortisol, boosting libido and reducing tension.

Panchakarma Detox

Uttar Basti (Ayurvedic vaginal therapy) – Medicated ghee/oil nourishes vaginal tissues.

Fertility & Libido Tea

Ingredients: Shatavari, Ashwagandha, saffron, cardamom, warm milk.
Effects: Enhances moisture and sexual vitality.
Modern Medical Solutions: Science-Backed Relief
Estrogen Therapy (Topical creams & vaginal rings for menopausal women).
Hyaluronic Acid-Based Lubricants (Mimics natural moisture).

Pelvic Floor Therapy (Exercises to relax vaginal muscles).

Omega-3 Supplements (Improves tissue hydration).
Conclusion: Reawakening Feminine Comfort & Confidence
Painful intimacy and dryness are not just physical challenges but deeply connected to a woman's hormonal health, emotions, and self-care. By embracing a holistic approach that blends Ayurvedic

wisdom with modern solutions, a woman can reclaim her pleasure, confidence, and intimate well-being.

"A nourished body blooms, just like a well-watered lotus in the warmth of the sun."

Chapter 15

FEMALE INFERTILITY

Introduction: The Sacred Creation of Life

In Ayurveda, a woman's ability to conceive is compared to a fertile field (Kshetra) where the seed (Shukra Dhatu) must be strong, the soil (Rasa Dhatu) must be nourished, and the environment (Agni & Doshas) must be balanced. When any of these elements are disturbed, infertility (Vandhyatva) occurs.

"ऋतुक्षेत्रं अम्बु बीजं संयोगात् गर्भसंभवः।"
चरक संहिता, चिकित्सा स्थान, 30.25
(For conception, proper timing (ovulation), a healthy uterus, nourishing fluids, and a strong seed are essential.)

Metaphor: The Blooming Tree of Fertility

Just as a tree flourishes with the right sunlight, water, and soil, a woman's reproductive system requires hormonal balance, nourishment, and emotional well-being to bear fruit.

Causes of Female Infertility: Ayurvedic & Modern Perspective
Ayurvedic Causes: Dosha Imbalances & Infertility
Vata Imbalance (Irregular Ovulation & Weak Implantation)
Symptoms: Dryness, scanty periods, anxiety, weight loss.
Causes: Stress, excessive exercise, late-night work, processed foods.
Remedies: Warm oil massage (Abhyanga), Ashwagandha, sesame oil.
Pitta Imbalance (Inflammation & Hormonal Issues)
Symptoms: Heavy bleeding, PCOS, endometriosis, excessive heat in the body.

Causes: Spicy foods, anger, excessive caffeine, smoking.
Remedies: Cooling herbs (Shatavari, Aloe Vera), coconut oil, meditation.
Kapha Imbalance (Blocked Fallopian Tubes & PCOS)
Symptoms: Obesity, slow metabolism, cystic ovaries, excessive mucus.
Causes: Sedentary lifestyle, excess dairy, emotional dullness.
Remedies: Light exercise, fenugreek seeds, dry massages.

"रक्तशुद्धौ प्रसन्नत्वं पौंसत्वं गर्भाशयस्थितिः।"
सुश्रुत संहिता, शरीर स्थान2.33

(healthy reproductive system ensures conception and sustains pregnancy.)

Modern Causes of Female Infertility

Hormonal Disorders (PCOS, thyroid imbalance, early menopause).
Structural Issues (Blocked fallopian tubes, fibroids, endometriosis).
Lifestyle Factors (Stress, smoking, alcohol, obesity).
Age & Genetics (Diminished ovarian reserve, chromosomal abnormalities).

Ayurvedic Panchakarma for Fertility Boosting

Panchakarma therapy detoxifies the reproductive system, balances hormones, and enhances fertility.
Vamana (Therapeutic Emesis) — Removes excess Kapha, helpful for PCOS.
Virechana (Purgation Therapy) — Detoxifies liver & balances Pitta for hormonal health.
Basti (Medicated Enema) — Regulates Vata, nourishes uterus & boosts egg quality.

Uttar Basti (Vaginal Oil Therapy) – Removes blockages, enhances uterine strength.
Nasya (Nasal Therapy) – Clears toxins affecting the reproductive hormones.

Case Study: Panchakarma Success in PCOS
Pooja, a 32-year-old woman, struggled with infertility due to irregular periods and ovarian cysts. After three months of Panchakarma (Virechana, Basti, Uttar Basti) and Ayurvedic herbs (Shatavari, Ashwagandha), her cycle regularized, her cysts shrank, and she conceived naturally.

Ayurvedic Herbs for Female Fertility

Shatavari – The Queen of Reproductive Health
Nourishes Shukra Dhatu, regulates estrogen, and enhances ovulation.
Ashwagandha – The Stress Reliever
Lowers cortisol, improves egg quality, and regulates cycles.
Gokshura – The Hormone Balancer
Strengthens ovaries, reduces PCOS symptoms, and enhances libido.
Pippali (Long Pepper) – The Uterine Cleanser
Detoxifies the uterus and boosts implantation success.

Saffron & Dry Fruits

Improves blood circulation and warmth for implantation.
Assisted Reproductive Technology (ART): Modern Science for Infertility
For women facing persistent infertility, ART solutions offer medical advancements to support conception.
Ovulation Induction (OI) – Hormonal treatment to stimulate egg production.

Intrauterine Insemination (IUI) – Direct sperm placement for better chances.
In Vitro Fertilization (IVF) – Lab-assisted fertilization of eggs & sperm.
Intracytoplasmic Sperm Injection (ICSI) – A refined IVF technique for male infertility.
Egg Freezing & Donor Eggs – For age-related infertility challenges.

Case Study: Ayurvedic Support for IVF Success
Nisha, a 35-year-old woman, had two failed IVF attempts due to thin endometrial lining and stress. She incorporated Panchakarma, Shatavari, and Ashwagandha for three months before her third IVF. This time, her endometrial thickness improved, her stress reduced, and she successfully conceived.

Conclusion: A Balanced Approach to Fertility
Infertility is not just a medical condition—it is a holistic concern involving physical, emotional, and lifestyle factors. By integrating Ayurvedic detox, herbal therapy, emotional well-being, and ART solutions, a woman can rekindle her reproductive strength and embrace the journey to motherhood.

"A nourished womb is like fertile soil—when cared for with love, patience, and wisdom, it blossoms into life."

Chapter 16

PCOS, HORMONES & SEXUAL HEALTH

Introduction: The Feminine Rhythm and Balance

A woman's body is a symphony of hormones, each playing a vital role in her health, energy, and sexuality. When this harmony is disturbed by Polycystic Ovary Syndrome (PCOS), it affects not just fertility but also emotional and sexual well-being.

Metaphor: The Broken Clock of Womanhood

Imagine the female body as a beautifully designed clock, where hormones are the gears ensuring smooth functioning. In PCOS, the gears (hormones) misalign, disrupting ovulation, metabolism, and libido. Ayurveda and holistic medicine aim to restore the clock's natural rhythm.

PCOS: Understanding the Root Cause
PCOS is not just an ovarian disorder—it is a metabolic, hormonal, and inflammatory condition affecting periods, weight, skin, fertility, and sexual health.

Ayurvedic Perspective: PCOS as a Tridoshic Disorder
PCOS arises from an imbalance of all three doshas:
Vata (Irregular periods, dryness, anxiety)
Pitta (Inflammation, acne, anger, heat in the body)
Kapha (Weight gain, lethargy, insulin resistance)

"दोषदूष्यसम्मूर्छनात् व्याधिनिष्पत्तिः।" चरक संहिता (चिकित्सा स्थान 30.26)
(When doshas accumulate and disturb bodily tissues, disease manifests.)

Modern Science: Key Hormonal Imbalances in PCOS
Excess Androgens → Irregular periods, facial hair (Hirsutism), acne.
Insulin Resistance → Weight gain, sugar cravings, Type-2 Diabetes risk.
Low Progesterone → Anxiety, poor sleep, infertility.
High Estrogen & Low SHBG → Water retention, mood swings, bloating.

PCOS & Sexual Health: The Unspoken Struggles

Women with PCOS often experience:
Low Libido – Hormonal imbalance leads to reduced sexual desire.
Vaginal Dryness & Painful Intercourse – Low estrogen affects lubrication.
Body Image Issues – Weight gain, acne, and hair loss impact self-esteem.
Emotional Disconnect – Anxiety, stress, and mood swings reduce intimacy.

Case Study: PCOS and Relationship Challenges
Megha, a 29-year-old woman, struggled with irregular cycles, excess weight, and low libido. Frustrated with failed treatments, she turned to Ayurveda. Through a regimen of Shatavari, Ashwagandha, oil massages (Abhyanga), and stress management, her cycle regularized, and intimacy in her marriage improved.
Holistic Healing: Ayurveda's Approach to PCOS & Sexual Health
Healing PCOS is about balancing hormones, reducing stress, and improving metabolic health through Ayurveda's dietary, herbal, detox, and lifestyle interventions.

1. Ayurvedic Detox: Panchakarma for PCOS
- Panchakarma is the gold standard for resetting the body.
- Virechana (Purgation Therapy) – Clears excess Pitta & regulates hormones.

- Basti (Medicated Enema) – Nourishes reproductive organs, balances Vata.
- Uttar Basti (Vaginal Therapy) – Improves uterine health & sexual wellness.
- Nasya (Nasal Therapy) – Clears toxins affecting the hormonal axis.

3. Ayurvedic Herbs for PCOS & Sexual Wellness

Shatavari – Regulates estrogen, boosts libido, improves lubrication.
Ashwagandha – Reduces cortisol, enhances mood & sexual stamina.
Gokshura – Boosts testosterone balance & sexual vitality.
Triphala – Detoxifies the gut, aiding metabolism.
Cinnamon & Fenugreek – Improves insulin sensitivity.
"स्त्रियः प्रियतमा लोके पुष्पिता कल्याणमुच्यते।"
अष्टांग हृदयम
(A nourished woman blossoms in health, joy, and well-being.)
Yoga & Breathwork: Restoring Feminine Energy
Butterfly Pose (Baddha Konasana) – Stimulates ovaries, increases blood flow.
Cobra Pose (Bhujangasana) – Opens pelvic region, balances hormones.
Deep Belly Breathing (Pranayama) – Reduces stress, improves libido.
Yoni Mudra – Strengthens reproductive energy & promotes intimacy.

Case Study: Yoga & Libido in PCOS
Anita, a 35-year-old with PCOS, struggled with painful intercourse and emotional disconnection. After six months of Yoga & Ayurvedic therapy, she reported increased confidence, better lubrication, and improved marital harmony.

Modern Treatments: When to Consider Medical Interventions?
If natural methods do not yield results, women may explore:
Hormonal Therapy (Birth Control Pills, Metformin, Spironolactone)
Fertility Treatments (Ovulation Induction, IVF)

Laser Hair Removal for Hirsutism

Integrative Case Study: Ayurveda + Modern Medicine for PCOS
Pallavi, a 32-year-old with PCOS & infertility, combined Ayurvedic Panchakarma with IVF preparation. She took Shatavari, Ashwagandha, & Gokshura along with her fertility treatment. Her third IVF cycle was successful, proving that an integrative approach works best.

Conclusion: Reclaiming Feminine Health Naturally
Healing PCOS is not just about treating symptoms—it's about restoring a woman's rhythm, sensuality, and inner glow. Ayurveda, Yoga, and a mindful lifestyle create a natural path to hormonal harmony and sexual wellness.

"A woman in balance is a goddess in her own right."

Chapter 17

MENOPAUSE & SEXUALITY

Introduction: The Second Spring of Womanhood
Menopause is often viewed as the end of youth, but in Ayurveda, it is seen as the beginning of wisdom and new vitality. Just as a river, after flowing turbulently, finds its calm yet deep course, a woman's energy shifts from creation to rejuvenation.

Metaphor: The Phoenix Rising

Imagine a woman's sexual energy as a Phoenix—not something that dies with menopause, but rather burns old limitations and rises stronger. With the right Ayurvedic practices and mindset, she can rediscover pleasure, intimacy, and a deep connection with herself.

Understanding Menopause & Sexual Changes

Menopause is the transition from the Pitta stage (fertility) to the Vata stage (wisdom and renewal). It brings hormonal shifts that can impact sexual health.

Ayurvedic Perspective: The Dosha Shift
Vata Aggravation → Dryness, anxiety, low libido.
Pitta Imbalance → Hot flashes, irritability, emotional outbursts.
Kapha Accumulation → Weight gain, lethargy, loss of enthusiasm.
"जरा जन्तूनां भवति स्वभावः।" चरक संहिता
(Aging is natural, but balance maintains health.)

Modern Science: The Hormonal Shift
Declining Estrogen & Testosterone → Lower libido, vaginal dryness.

Decreased Oxytocin & Dopamine → Reduced emotional connection.
Increased Cortisol → Stress, irritability, and fatigue.

Common Sexual Concerns After Menopause

Vaginal Dryness & Painful Intercourse – Due to declining estrogen levels.
Reduced Libido – Lower testosterone and emotional disconnection.
Body Image Issues – Weight changes and skin aging affect confidence.
Emotional Distance in Relationships – Mood swings and stress impact intimacy.

Case Study: Rediscovering Passion at 50
Suman, a 52-year-old teacher, felt disconnected from her husband after menopause. She experienced painful intimacy, mood swings, and low self-esteem. Through Ayurvedic herbs, Yoga, and mindful intimacy practices, she regained her confidence, and her marital bond deepened.

Ayurvedic Solutions for Menopausal Sexual Wellness

1. Panchakarma: Detoxifying for Rejuvenation

Menopause marks the body's natural aging process, and Panchakarma (Ayurvedic detox) helps restore vitality.
Virechana (Purgation Therapy) – Removes excess Pitta, reducing hot flashes.
Basti (Medicated Enema) – Balances Vata, nourishes reproductive organs.
Nasya (Nasal Therapy) – Clears mental fog, improves mood and energy.

2. Ayurvedic Herbs for Passion & Vitality

Shatavari (Queen of Herbs) – Restores feminine energy & lubrication.
Ashwagandha – Reduces stress, boosts libido & stamina.
Kapikacchu (Mucuna Pruriens) – Increases dopamine, enhancing pleasure.
Vidarikand – Strengthens reproductive tissues & vaginal health.
Triphala – Supports digestion and prevents bloating.

"शतावरी हिमं श्रेष्ठं स्तन्य शुक्र बल प्रदम्।"
अष्टांग हृदयम

(Shatavari is cooling, nourishes reproductive tissues, and strengthens vitality.)

3. Diet: Foods to Boost Libido & Hormonal Balance

Sesame Seeds & Ghee – Lubricates tissues, improving vaginal health.
Figs, Dates & Almonds – Aphrodisiac foods that enhance energy.
Fenugreek & Ashwagandha Tea – Boosts estrogen & testosterone naturally.
Turmeric & Cinnamon – Reduces inflammation, enhancing pleasure.
Yoga & Breathwork: Awakening Feminine Energy
Best Yoga Poses for Menopausal Sexual Wellness
Butterfly Pose (Baddha Konasana) – Stimulates ovaries, improving blood flow.
Cobra Pose (Bhujangasana) – Opens the heart chakra, enhancing intimacy.
Cat-Cow (Marjaryasana-Bitilasana) – Increases pelvic flexibility.
Pelvic Tilts & Kegels – Strengthens vaginal muscles, improving pleasure.
Pranayama (Breathwork) for Sexual Vitality

Bhramari (Humming Bee Breath) – Relieves stress, enhances feminine energy.
Nadi Shodhana (Alternate Nostril Breathing) – Balances hormones & mood.

Case Study: Yoga & Sensuality in the 40s
Anita, a 48-year-old executive, noticed a drop in libido and vaginal dryness. She started a daily Yoga and breathwork routine, which improved circulation, emotional connection, and pleasure during intimacy.

Modern Medical Interventions: When to Consider Them?
Hormone Replacement Therapy (HRT) – For severe estrogen deficiency.
Vaginal Estrogen Creams – Helps with lubrication and dryness.
Pelvic Physical Therapy – For improving muscle strength.

Integrative Case Study: Ayurveda + Modern Medicine
Pallavi, 55, combined Ayurvedic herbs with HRT and saw remarkable improvements in mood, sexual health, and energy levels. A combined approach often yields the best results.

Rediscovering Intimacy: Mindful Connection with Your Partner
Ayurvedic Body Massage (Abhyanga) – Nourishes tissues, enhances sensuality.
Tantric Practices – Slow, mindful intimacy to enhance pleasure.
Oxytocin-Boosting Activities – Dancing, laughing, and cuddling together.

Quote:
"Love does not fade with age; it deepens like a well-nourished tree."

Conclusion: Menopause is Not an End—It's a New Beginning

Sexuality after 40 is about redefining pleasure, embracing self-love, and nourishing intimacy. With Ayurveda, menopause becomes a journey of self-discovery and empowerment.
"A woman's body is not meant to wither with age, but to bloom in wisdom."

SECTION 4

HOLISTIC THERAPIES FOR SEXUAL WELLNESS

Chapter 18

VAJIKARANA CHIKITSA OF AYURVEDA

1. Introduction to Vajikarana Chikitsa

Vajikarana (वाजीकरण) is one of the eight branches of Ayurveda that deals with sexual health, vitality, and reproductive wellness. It is derived from the Sanskrit word 'Vaji' (वाजी), meaning horse, symbolizing strength and virility.

"वाजीकरण द्रव्याणि स्युः शुक्रवर्धन हेतवः।
प्रजनन सुखोदारकाः शरीर बलवर्धनाः ॥"
चरक संहिता (चिकित्सा स्थान 1.17)
(Vajikarana therapies enhance reproductive fluids, promote pleasure, and increase physical strength.)

2. The Importance of Sexual Rejuvenation in Ayurveda

Sexual energy (Shukra Dhatu) is considered the essence of Ojas (vital immunity and longevity factor). Ayurveda states that balanced sexual health leads to overall well-being, while its depletion leads to fatigue, weakness, and mental stress.

Metaphor: "Just as a lamp needs oil to burn brightly, the body needs healthy Shukra Dhatu for energy and vitality."

Case Study: A 42-year-old businessman suffering from chronic stress and declining libido regained vitality after following a Vajikarana regimen including Ashwagandha, Shatavari, and specific lifestyle modifications.

3. Vajikarana Herbs and Aphrodisiacs

Ayurveda prescribes potent herbs and formulations for sexual rejuvenation:

A. Key Vajikarana Herbs

- Ashwagandha (Withania Somnifera) — Known as "Indian Ginseng," it enhances stamina and stress resistance.
- Shatavari (Asparagus Racemosus) — "Queen of Herbs," supports female reproductive health.
- Kapikacchu (Mucuna Pruriens) — Boosts libido and sperm quality.
- Gokshura (Tribulus Terrestris) — Increases testosterone and energy.
- Safed Musli (Chlorophytum Borivilianum) — Powerful aphrodisiac and sperm enhancer.

B. Ayurvedic Aphrodisiac Formulations

Vrishya Ghrita (medicated ghee for virility)
Makardhwaj Rasayana (gold-based rejuvenative)
Kameshwar Modaka (herbal confection for enhanced libido)

4. Diet & Lifestyle in Vajikarana

Diet plays a crucial role in sexual health. Ayurveda prescribes a Sattvic diet with nuts, seeds, dairy, ghee, and wholesome grains.

"घृतं दध्ना पयः सक्तुः शालि मुद्गा यवस्तथा।
वृष्याणि च वृष्यं च वर्जयेत् कर्मदुष्टिदम्॥"
अष्टांग हृदयम (सूत्रस्थान 11.10)
(Ghee, milk, barley, and green gram enhance virility, whereas stress and unhealthy habits deplete it.)

Metaphor: "A well-nourished body is like a well-watered tree—bearing strong roots (health), fragrant flowers (energy), and sweet fruits (pleasure)."

5. Vajikarana Therapy: Classical Ayurvedic Treatments

Ayurveda prescribes Panchakarma-based detox before Vajikarana therapy:
Abhyanga (Oil Massage) – Enhances circulation and nervous system function.
Swedana (Herbal Steam Therapy) – Clears toxins from tissues.
Basti (Medicated Enema) – Balances Vata Dosha affecting sexual health.
Shirodhara (Oil Pouring on Forehead) – Reduces stress-related impotence.

Case Study: A 35-year-old IT professional with performance anxiety saw significant improvement after a Panchakarma detox followed by Vajikarana Rasayanas.

6. Psychological Aspects of Vajikarana

Ayurveda emphasizes mental and emotional well-being as essential for sexual health.
Bhava (Emotion) Therapy: Love, affection, and relaxation are essential.
Meditation & Yoga: Practices like Vajroli Mudra, Baddha Konasana, and Pranayama enhance Ojas.

"युक्ताहारविहारस्य युक्तचेष्ट्स्य कर्मसु।
युक्तस्वप्नावबोधस्य योगो भवति दुःखहा ॥" भगवत गीता (6.16)
(Balanced diet, routine, and sleep lead to a healthy body and mind.)

7. Modern Research & Relevance of Vajikarana

Recent studies have validated Ayurvedic aphrodisiacs:
Ashwagandha improves sperm quality and testosterone levels.
Shatavari boosts estrogen and fertility in women.
Tribulus Terrestris increases libido and erectile function.

Case Study: A clinical trial on Ashwagandha at Banaras Hindu University showed a 30% increase in sperm count after 90 days of usage.

8. Conclusion: Vajikarana is not just about sexual performance but about holistic well-being, vitality, and longevity. Integrating Ayurvedic herbs, therapies, diet, and mental wellness practices helps in sustaining a fulfilling and healthy life.

Chapter 19

YOGA & MEDITATION FOR SEXUAL HEALTH

1. Introduction: The Union of Mind & Body in Sexual Well-being
Sexual health in Ayurveda and Yoga is not just about physical pleasure but a harmonious balance of body, mind, and spirit. Yoga and meditation strengthen the Shukra Dhatu (reproductive tissue), enhance Ojas (vital energy), and regulate the Prana (life force energy), leading to longevity and vitality.

"सुखायुः कामार्थसिद्धिर्व्यधिक्षेमाय शरीरम्।
तदर्थं यत्नतः शश्वत् शरीरम् अनुपालयेत्॥"
Charaka Samhita (Sutrasthana 30.26)
(A healthy body ensures pleasure, success, and protection from diseases; hence, one should maintain it with care.)

2. How Yoga & Meditation Improve Sexual Health

Yoga and meditation enhance sexual function by:
Regulating hormones (testosterone, estrogen, dopamine)
Reducing stress & anxiety, which cause erectile dysfunction and low libido
Improving circulation to the reproductive organs
Enhancing stamina & flexibility for better performance
Balancing the nervous system, ensuring better arousal and satisfaction

Metaphor: "Just as a river must flow smoothly without obstacles to reach the ocean, the energy within the body must flow freely for a fulfilling sexual life."

3. Yogic Practices for Sexual Vitality

A. Asanas (Postures) for Sexual Health

The following postures increase blood circulation, stimulate endocrine glands, and strengthen pelvic muscles:
Bhujangasana (Cobra Pose) – Enhances blood flow to the reproductive organs.
Ustrasana (Camel Pose) – Opens the heart and stimulates hormonal balance.
Baddha Konasana (Butterfly Pose) – Improves flexibility and circulation in pelvic muscles.
Dhanurasana (Bow Pose) – Stimulates sexual energy and relieves fatigue.
Vajroli Mudra (Thunderbolt Gesture) – Increases sexual control and stamina.

"वज्रोली नाम मुद्रायं साधनं परमं स्मृतम्।
योगिनामपि मुख्यस्य सिद्धिर्भवति निश्चितम्॥"
Yoga Pradipika (Chapter 1, Verse 66)
(Vajroli Mudra is a supreme practice; it grants mastery over sexual energy and enhances vitality.)

4. Pranayama (Breathing Techniques) for Sexual Energy

Controlled breathing helps in enhancing Prana (life force energy) and improves endurance.
Nadi Shodhana (Alternate Nostril Breathing) – Balances hormones and mental clarity.
Bhastrika (Bellows Breath) – Increases stamina and boosts testosterone.
Kapalabhati (Skull-Shining Breath) – Detoxifies reproductive organs.

Case Study: A 38-year-old male suffering from premature ejaculation practiced Bhastrika and Nadi Shodhana for 3 months, experiencing improved control and confidence in intimacy.

5. Meditation for Sexual Rejuvenation

Meditation reduces stress, improves concentration, and deepens intimacy in relationships.

A. Types of Meditation for Sexual Health

Mindfulness Meditation — Increases awareness of sensations and enhances arousal.
Kundalini Meditation — Awakens dormant sexual energy (Kundalini Shakti).
Trataka (Candle Gazing) — Improves focus and enhances intimate connection.

"उद्धरेदात्मनाऽत्मानं नात्मानमवसादयेत्।
आत्मैव ह्यात्मनो बन्धुरात्मैव रिपुरात्मनः ॥"
Bhagavad Gita (6.5):
(A person must elevate himself through his mind and not degrade himself, for the mind is both a friend and an enemy.)

Case Study: A 45-year-old woman suffering from low libido and emotional disconnect practiced mindfulness meditation for 6 weeks, leading to enhanced intimacy and emotional bonding with her partner.

6. Bandhas & Mudras for Sexual Control

A. Bandhas (Energy Locks) to Channel Sexual Energy
Mula Bandha (Root Lock) — Strengthens pelvic muscles, preventing premature ejaculation.

Uddiyana Bandha (Abdominal Lock) – Stimulates energy flow to sexual organs.

B. Mudras (Hand Gestures) for Sexual Vitality

Yoni Mudra – Enhances feminine energy and reproductive health.
Shakti Mudra – Strengthens libido and balances hormones.

7.   The Role of Celibacy & Brahmacharya in Longevity

Ayurveda and Yoga emphasize Brahmacharya (moderation in sexual activity) to preserve Ojas. Excessive indulgence weakens energy levels, while balanced sexual activity enhances vitality.

"ब्रह्मचर्येण तपसा देवर्षित्वं प्रपद्यते।
इन्द्रियाणां निरोधेन अमर्त्यत्वं आप्नुयात् सदा॥"
Manusmriti (2.91)
(By practicing celibacy and self-restraint, one attains divine energy and longevity.)
Metaphor: "A candle that burns too fast soon fades, but one that burns steadily lasts longer."

Case   Study: A   50-year-old   practitioner   of   controlled Brahmacharya reported enhanced physical strength, sharper intellect, and improved relationships.

8.   Scientific Research on Yoga, Meditation & Sexual Health

Studies show that practicing yoga for 12 weeks increases testosterone levels and improves erectile function.
Mindfulness meditation has been found to reduce performance anxiety and increase sexual satisfaction.

Case Study: Harvard Medical School found that women who practiced yoga regularly experienced a 20% increase in sexual desire and satisfaction.

9. **Conclusion:** Yoga and meditation offer a natural, sustainable way to enhance sexual health, boost longevity, and improve overall well-being. Through consistent practice, one can awaken inner vitality, deepen intimate connections, and live a more fulfilling life.

"शरीरेन्द्रियसत्त्वात्मसंयोगो धारि जीवितम्।
नित्यगः सर्वथा सन्निवृत्तस्य तु तद्ध्रुवम्॥"
Sushruta Samhita (Sutrasthana 15.48)

Chapter 20

TANTRIC PRACTICES & SEXUAL ENERGY

1. Introduction: The Sacred Power of Sexual Energy
In Tantra, sexual energy (Shakti) is not just a means of pleasure but a transformative force that leads to higher consciousness and spiritual awakening. The union of Shiva (pure consciousness) and Shakti (dynamic energy) represents the ultimate realization of divine potential within.

"कन्दर्पकोटिलावण्यं शक्तो यत्र प्रपूर्यते।
तत्रैव शक्तिसन्दोहः शिवमावेष्टयत्यधः॥"
Vijnana Bhairava Tantra (Verse 69)
(When the energy of millions of Cupids is awakened within, it unites with the divine consciousness, leading to ultimate bliss.)

4. Understanding Sexual Energy in Tantra

Tantra views Kundalini Shakti as the dormant sexual energy coiled at the base of the spine. By awakening and directing this energy through Tantric practices, one experiences:
Heightened pleasure & spiritual ecstasy
Strengthened vital force (Ojas & Tejas)
Prolonged youthfulness & longevity
Deepened intimacy & emotional connection

Metaphor: "Just as fire, when controlled, can cook food and provide warmth, but when uncontrolled, can destroy—sexual energy, when mastered, leads to enlightenment; when misused, leads to depletion."

3. Tantric Yoga for Sexual Energy Enhancement
Certain Asanas (postures) and Bandhas (energy locks) help channel and refine sexual energy.

A. Asanas for Strengthening Sexual Vitality

Ashwini Mudra (Horse Gesture) — Contracts pelvic muscles, increasing control over sexual energy.
Ustrasana (Camel Pose) — Opens heart chakra and increases libido.
Viparita Karani (Legs-up-the-wall Pose) — Enhances reproductive health and stamina.
Bhujangasana (Cobra Pose) — Stimulates Kundalini awakening.
Mula Bandha (Root Lock) — Controls ejaculation and directs sexual energy upwards.

"मूलबन्धः सदा कार्यो युवानं योगिनां प्रिये।
आयुष्यं बलमासां वै बृंहणं शुभदायकम्॥"
Hatha Yoga Pradipika (3.5)
(Practicing Mula Bandha preserves youth, strengthens vitality, and enhances life energy.)

Case Study: A 40-year-old man suffering from low libido practiced Mula Bandha and Viparita Karani for three months, reporting increased stamina and deeper connection with his partner.

5. The Role of Pranayama & Mantras in Tantric Sexual Energy

Breath control and sound vibrations help harness and channel sexual energy.

A. Pranayama for Sexual Energy

Nadi Shodhana (Alternate Nostril Breathing) — Balances Shiva (masculine) and Shakti (feminine) energies.
Bhastrika (Bellows Breath) — Boosts testosterone and libido.
Ujjayi Pranayama (Victorious Breath) — Heightens sensory awareness and prolongs pleasure.

B. Mantras for Awakening Sexual Energy

Kleem Mantra ("Kleem") – Activates sexual attraction and magnetism.
Shakti Mantra ("Om Aim Hreem Kleem Chamundaye Vichche") – Enhances feminine energy.
Shiva-Shakti Mantra ("Om Namah Shivaya") – Balances masculine and feminine forces.

"उद्धरेदात्मनाऽत्मानं नात्मानमवसादयेत्।
आत्मैव ह्यात्मनो बन्धुरात्मैव रिपुरात्मनः॥"
Bhagavad Gita (6.5):

(One must elevate the self through the mind, as the mind can be both a friend and an enemy.)

Case Study: A 35-year-old woman practiced Nadi Shodhana and Kleem Mantra for six weeks, experiencing heightened intimacy and self-confidence.

6. The Role of Kundalini Awakening in Tantra

Kundalini energy is the coiled serpent energy at the base of the spine. When awakened, it rises through the chakras, transforming raw sexual energy into spiritual enlightenment.

A. Chakras & Sexual Energy Flow

Muladhara (Root Chakra) – Governs primal sexual energy.
Swadhisthana (Sacral Chakra) – Enhances creativity and passion.
Manipura (Solar Plexus Chakra) – Transmutes sexual energy into confidence.
Anahata (Heart Chakra) – Deepens emotional intimacy.
Vishuddha (Throat Chakra) – Enhances communication in relationships.

Ajna (Third Eye Chakra) — Increases spiritual perception in intimacy.
Sahasrara (Crown Chakra) — Leads to divine ecstasy.

Metaphor: "A river flowing freely nourishes life; when blocked, it creates stagnation. Similarly, blocked energy in the chakras leads to sexual frustration, while free-flowing energy leads to divine bliss."

Case Study: A 50-year-old couple engaged in Tantra meditation and Kundalini Yoga, leading to renewed passion and spiritual bonding in their relationship.

7. Tantric Rituals for Sexual Energy Mastery

A. Maithuna: The Sacred Union

Maithuna (Tantric lovemaking) is not just physical but a ritual of energy exchange leading to divine unity.
Prolonged Eye Contact — Enhances intimacy and spiritual connection.
Slow, Conscious Breathing — Syncs energies of both partners.
Yab-Yum Position — Represents the union of Shiva and Shakti.

"नास्ति मैथुनमानन्दमन्यत्संसारसंस्थितम्।
यत्र शक्तिर्विलीनास्यात्तत्र शिवात्मता स्थिता॥"
Kaulajnananirnaya Tantra
(There is no greater bliss than sacred union, where Shakti dissolves and Shiva manifests.)

Case Study: A newlywed couple practiced Maithuna with conscious breathing and experienced deeper emotional bonding and heightened intimacy.

8. The Power of Celibacy & Energy Conservation (Brahmacharya in Tantra)

While Tantra teaches sexual energy enhancement, it also emphasizes energy conservation (Brahmacharya) for spiritual growth.

A. Benefits of Energy Conservation

Enhances mental clarity & creativity
Increases physical stamina & vitality
Strengthens spiritual consciousness

Metaphor: "A lamp burns brighter when oil is conserved, just as a person thrives when vital energy is preserved and directed."

"ब्रह्मचर्येण तपसा देवर्षित्वं प्रपद्यते।
इन्द्रियाणां निरोधेन अमृतत्वं आप्नुयात् सदा॥"
Manusmriti (2.91)
(Through celibacy and self-restraint, one attains divine energy and longevity.)

Case Study: A 60-year-old monk practicing Brahmacharya and Kundalini meditation reported extraordinary health and mental sharpness.

9. Scientific Research on Tantra & Sexual Energy

Studies show that Tantra practitioners experience better sexual satisfaction and emotional bonding.
Harvard research confirms that mindful sexuality enhances relationship satisfaction and reduces stress.

9. Conclusion: Tantric practices offer a sacred path to harness and transform sexual energy for pleasure, vitality, and spiritual enlightenment. Whether through yoga, breathwork, mantras, or rituals, Tantra teaches the art of balancing desire with divinity, leading to profound inner fulfillment.

Chapter 21

ACUPRESSURE & MARMA THERAPY

1. Introduction: Awakening the Body's Hidden Energy
Acupressure and Marma Therapy, two ancient healing sciences, work by stimulating vital energy points in the body to restore balance, enhance vitality, and rejuvenate the senses. In Ayurveda and Traditional Chinese Medicine (TCM), sexual desire (Kama Shakti) is deeply linked to Prana (life force) and the health of the body's energy meridians (Nadis).

"वाजीकरणानां श्रेष्ठं मारुतं स्थापनं परम्।
तत्र श्रृंगारसंयुक्तं बलमिन्द्रियवर्धनम्॥"
Charaka Samhita (Chikitsa Sthana 30.26)
(The supreme aphrodisiac is the proper balance of Vata; it restores passion, strength, and sensory vigor.)

2. Understanding Marma & Acupressure for Desire Enhancement

Marma therapy (Ayurvedic acupressure) and TCM acupressure target vital points in the body to:
Stimulate libido and sexual vitality
Improve blood circulation to reproductive organs
Balance hormones linked to desire
Enhance emotional intimacy and well-being

Metaphor: "Just as pressing the right keys on a musical instrument creates a perfect melody, stimulating the right points on the body awakens dormant sexual energy."

4. Key Acupressure & Marma Points for Enhancing Desire

By pressing or massaging these points, one can restore sexual energy and enhance intimacy.

A. Marma Points in Ayurveda

- Basti Marma (Lower Abdomen, Bladder Point) – Stimulates sexual energy and enhances reproductive function.
- Nabhi Marma (Navel Center) – Strengthens Prana and digestive fire, linked to virility.
- Hridaya Marma (Heart Center) – Opens emotional blockages and deepens intimacy.
- Madhya Marma (Perineum, Base of Spine) – Awakens dormant sexual energy (Kundalini).
- Apanga Marma (Temple Region) – Stimulates desire by balancing mind-body energy.

B. Acupressure Points from TCM

CV6 (Qi Hai / Sea of Energy) – Lower Abdomen
Boosts sexual stamina and libido
Increases vital energy (Qi or Prana)
Press firmly for 1-2 minutes daily
SP6 (San Yin Jiao / Three Yin Crossing) – Inner Ankle
Balances reproductive hormones
Enhances sexual sensitivity in women
Massage gently before intimacy
GV4 (Ming Men / Gate of Life) – Lower Back
Rejuvenates kidney energy, the foundation of sexual vitality
Improves male virility and sperm health
LV3 (Tai Chong / Great Surge) – Foot between First Two Toes
Regulates liver energy, reducing stress-induced low libido
Enhances emotional connection in relationships
PC8 (Lao Gong / Palace of Toil) – Center of Palm

Stimulates passion and heart energy
Enhances tactile sensitivity during intimacy

Case Study: A 45-year-old man with low libido practiced daily acupressure on Qi Hai (CV6) and Ming Men (GV4) for three months and experienced renewed vitality and emotional intimacy in his marriage.

5.   The Role of Prana & Qi in Sexual Desire

In Ayurveda, sexual energy (Ojas) is the refined essence of Prana. In TCM, Jing (vital essence) governs reproductive health. Both systems emphasize:
Strong kidneys (Adrenal health) for sexual potency
Balanced heart energy for emotional bonding
Free-flowing energy (Nadis/Meridians) for pleasure and longevity

"ओजो धातुः परं श्रेष्ठं शरीरस्य परिग्रहः।
वीर्यं शरीरसंयोगं प्रजननार्थं संस्थितम्॥"
Sushruta Samhita (Sharira Sthana 4.30)
(Ojas is the supreme essence of life; it fuels sexual vigor and ensures procreation.)
Metaphor: "Just as a river nourishes the land when its flow is unblocked, desire flourishes when Prana flows freely through the body's energy channels."

6.   Marma Therapy & Acupressure Massage Techniques

Daily self-massage (Abhyanga) with aphrodisiac oils enhances the effects of Marma therapy.

A.   Oil Massage for Libido Boost

Ashwagandha Oil – Rejuvenates vitality and calms the mind.
Shatavari Oil – Enhances female desire and hormonal balance.

Clove & Cinnamon Oil – Stimulates blood circulation to reproductive organs.

B. Acupressure Massage Routine

Warm oil and gently press Nabhi Marma (navel center) for 1 minute.
Massage Hridaya Marma (heart center) with circular motions.
Press CV6 (Qi Hai) below the navel to stimulate sexual energy.
Massage LV3 (Tai Chong) on the foot to relieve stress.

Case Study: A 38-year-old woman experiencing low desire used Shatavari oil and daily acupressure on SP6 and Nabhi Marma for two months, reporting increased arousal and emotional fulfillment.

7. Emotional & Mental Blocks in Desire

Releasing Trauma through Marma Therapy
Sexual energy can be blocked by past trauma, stress, or emotional wounds. Marma therapy helps clear these blockages by:
Activating the Hridaya Marma (Heart Energy Center) to release emotional pain

Massaging Ajna Marma (Third Eye) to dissolve mental stress
Stimulating Apanga Marma (Temple Point) for mood enhancement

"मनोमात्रं जगत्सर्वं मनः कल्पितबन्धनम्।
मनः प्रभवति व्याधौ मनोमात्रं सुखप्रदम्॥"
Yoga Vasistha (3.16.28)
(The world is a creation of the mind; suffering and pleasure both originate from it.)

Metaphor: "Just as a blocked dam prevents water from reaching the fields, unresolved emotions block desire from flourishing."

Case Study: A 50-year-old woman with suppressed trauma experienced renewed passion after a month of Marma therapy on Hridaya (Heart) and Ajna (Third Eye) points, combined with guided meditation.

7. Scientific Research on Acupressure & Marma Therapy for Desire Enhancement

A 2017 study in the Journal of Acupuncture Research found that acupressure on CV6 and SP6 significantly improved libido in both men and women.
Ayurvedic Marma therapy research suggests that Hridaya Marma stimulation enhances oxytocin (the bonding hormone), improving intimacy.
Clinical trials on Acupuncture and Marma Therapy have shown improved testosterone levels, vaginal lubrication, and emotional bonding.

8. **Conclusion**: Acupressure and Marma Therapy provide a powerful, natural way to enhance sexual energy, restore balance, and deepen emotional connection. By stimulating key energy points, one can awaken passion, improve hormonal health, and rejuvenate intimacy.

"आनन्दं ब्रह्मणो रूपम्, आनन्दं ब्रह्मणः कर्म।
आनन्देनैव कल्पते, परमानन्दमाप्नुयात्॥"
Brihadaranyaka Upanishad (6.4.3)

Chapter 22

HERBS & SUPERFOODS FOR SEXUAL VITALITY

1. Introduction: The Power of Nature in Enhancing Sexual Vitality
Sexual vitality in Ayurveda is closely linked to Ojas (vital essence), Shukra Dhatu (reproductive tissue), and Prana (life force energy). Certain herbs and superfoods act as Vajikarana (aphrodisiacs), which:

Enhance libido and stamina
Improve hormonal balance

"वाजीकरणानां श्रेष्ठानि शुक्रवर्धनकारणम्।
प्रजननसुखोत्पत्तिः शरीरबलवर्धनम्॥"
Charaka Samhita (Chikitsa Sthana 1.1.7)
(Vajikarana herbs increase reproductive fluids, promote pleasure, and strengthen the body.)
Metaphor: "Just as fuel strengthens a fire, the right herbs nourish and enhance sexual energy."

2. Ashwagandha (Withania Somnifera): The King of Vajikarana Herbs

- Benefits for Sexual Health
- Increases testosterone and sperm count
- Reduces stress and performance anxiety
- Enhances stamina and energy levels

"बालाद्वया तु कामार्थी वृष्यं बल्यं रसायनम्।
वातश्लेष्मविनाशाय शक्तिदं शुक्रलं परम्॥"
Bhavaprakasha Nighantu

(Ashwagandha is an aphrodisiac, rejuvenator, and strength-enhancer; it balances Vata and Kapha and increases reproductive fluids.)

Case Study: A 42-year-old male experiencing low libido and chronic fatigue took 5 grams of Ashwagandha powder daily with warm milk. After three months, he reported:
 Improved energy levels
 Increased sexual stamina
Better stress management

4. **Shatavari (Asparagus Racemosus): The Queen of Feminine Vitality**

   - Benefits for Women's Sexual Health
   - Enhances fertility and libido
   - Balances hormones and estrogen levels
   - Increases vaginal lubrication

Case Study: A 35-year-old woman suffering from low libido and irregular cycles consumed Shatavari Kalpa (powder mixed with milk) for two months. Results:

   - Enhanced sexual desire
   - Hormonal balance restored
   - Increased natural lubrication

5. **Safed Musli (Chlorophytum Borivilianum)**

- The Natural Viagra
- Benefits for Sexual Vitality
- Improves erectile function and sperm quality
- Increases libido and stamina
- Strengthens male reproductive health

- Traditional Ayurvedic Use
- Often used in Makardhwaj Rasayana, a rejuvenation therapy for sexual vigor.

Consumed as a decoction with milk and honey.

Metaphor: "Like fertile soil nourishes a strong tree, Safed Musli nourishes and strengthens reproductive power."

Case Study: A 50-year-old male struggling with erectile dysfunction took Safed Musli capsules for three months, reporting:

Increased firmness and duration

Higher sperm count

Improved overall vitality

6. Gokshura (Tribulus Terrestris)

The Testosterone Booster

Benefits for Sexual Health

Boosts testosterone levels naturally

Increases libido and sexual performance

Improves kidney function, which is linked to Shukra Dhatu

"गोक्षुरं शुक्रजननं वातपित्तकफप्रशमनम्।
वृष्यं बलवर्धनं च शरीरमायुष्यं तथा॥"

Bhavaprakasha Nighantu

(Gokshura enhances sperm production, balances all three doshas, increases strength, and promotes longevity.)

Case Study: A 28-year-old athlete with low testosterone supplemented with Gokshura extract for 60 days and experienced:

- Higher energy levels
- Increased muscle mass

- Enhanced sexual desire

6. Mucuna Pruriens (Kapikacchu): The Dopamine Enhancer
Benefits for Sexual Vitality

Increases dopamine levels, enhancing pleasure and performance
Improves sperm count and motility
Reduces stress-related libido loss

Traditional Use

Mixed with Ashwagandha for a powerful Vajikarana effect.
Metaphor: "Like a well-oiled machine runs smoothly, Kapikacchu ensures smooth functioning of the reproductive system."

Case Study: A 38-year-old man with low motivation and sexual exhaustion consumed Kapikacchu powder daily for three months and reported:
- Increased drive and motivation
- Enhanced sexual pleasure
- Improved sperm quality

7. Superfoods for Sexual Health & Longevity

Alongside herbs, certain superfoods naturally boost sexual energy:

A. Almonds & Walnuts

Rich in Zinc & Omega-3, essential for testosterone production.
Enhances blood circulation to reproductive organs.

B. Dates & Figs

Natural aphrodisiacs used in Arabian cultures.
Improve energy levels and libido.

C. Dark Chocolate

Contains phenylethylamine, which boosts mood and arousal.
Increases dopamine levels for enhanced pleasure.

D. Saffron & Nutmeg

Traditional libido enhancers in Ayurvedic and Unani medicine.
Saffron is known as a "natural Viagra".

Case Study: A 32-year-old woman included dates, saffron-infused milk, and almonds in her diet for six weeks. She reported:
Higher libido
Improved emotional intimacy
Reduced stress levels

8. Combining Herbs & Superfoods: The Ultimate Vajikarana Formula
For maximum effect, a combination of these herbs and foods can be taken in the form of:
Herbal milk tonics (Ashwagandha + Shatavari + Saffron in warm milk)
Chyawanprash (Ayurvedic jam) containing multiple aphrodisiac herbs
Ghee-based formulations like Vrishya Ghrita

9. Conclusion: The Holistic Path to Sexual Wellness
Sexual vitality is not just about performance but holistic health. Ayurveda teaches that a well-nourished body, balanced hormones, and a calm mind lead to a fulfilling intimate life.

SECTION 5

LIFESTYLE, DIET & MINDSET FOR SEX

Chapter 23

DAILY & SEASONAL ROUTINES FOR SEXUAL HEALTH

Sexual health is an essential pillar of overall well-being. Ayurveda considers it a reflection of physical, mental, and spiritual balance. Just as a plant needs the right amount of sunlight, water, and nutrients, our sexual health thrives on a disciplined lifestyle, proper nutrition, and seasonal adaptation.
Quote:
"When diet is wrong, medicine is of no use. When diet is correct, medicine is of no need." – Ayurvedic Proverb

1. Daily Routine (Dinacharya) for Sexual Vitality

Ayurveda recommends following a structured daily regimen to maintain Ojas (vital energy), which directly influences sexual health.
Morning Rituals (Brahma Muhurta – 4:30 to 6:00 AM)
Wake up early (Brahma Muhurta) – Enhances energy, clarity, and hormonal balance.

"कराग्रे वसते लक्ष्मीः करमध्ये सरस्वती।
करमूले तु गोविन्दः प्रभाते करदर्शनम्॥"
(This shloka reminds us of divinity in our hands and the importance of righteous actions.)
Drink lukewarm water with honey or Triphala – Detoxifies and balances digestion.
Oil pulling & tongue scraping – Removes toxins and enhances oral health.

Exercise & Yoga for Sexual Energy

Surya Namaskar (Sun Salutation) – Improves circulation and hormonal balance.
Mool Bandha & Ashwini Mudra – Strengthen pelvic muscles and enhance sexual performance.
Pranayama (Breathwork) – Boosts testosterone and energy levels.

Case Study: A 42-year-old man suffering from premature ejaculation incorporated Mool Bandha, Kapalbhati, and a Satvik diet into his routine. Within three months, he noticed a 60% improvement in endurance and overall sexual satisfaction.

Diet & Nutrition for Sexual Strength

Breakfast: Almonds, dates, figs, and saffron-infused milk – These nourish Shukra Dhatu (reproductive tissue).
Lunch: Balanced meal with ghee, seasonal vegetables, and whole grains.
Dinner: Light, warm food. Avoid heavy, fried, and processed foods.

Metaphor: "A strong sexual drive is like a well-lit lamp. If the oil (nutrition) is pure, the flame (vitality) burns brightly."

Evening & Night Rituals

Abhyanga (Self-Massage with Herbal Oils) – Reduces stress and strengthens the nervous system.
Shatavari & Ashwagandha Infused Milk – Boosts libido and reproductive health.
Early Sleep (Before 10 PM) – Ensures melatonin secretion and reproductive hormone regulation.

Shloka on Sleep:

"Ratri swasthya rakshartham nidra shreshtha upacharyate."
(Sleep is the best medicine for good health.)

2.   **Seasonal Routines (Ritucharya) for Sexual Health**

Just as nature changes, our body adapts to different seasons.
Ayurveda emphasizes modifying lifestyle and diet accordingly.
Spring (Vasanta Ritu – March to May)
Cleansing: Detox with herbal teas (Triphala, Neem).
Herbs: Gokshura and Kaunch Beej enhance stamina.
Exercise: Moderate workouts to prevent Kapha accumulation.

Metaphor: "Spring is like adolescence; energy is abundant, but direction is key."
Summer (Grishma Ritu – June to August)
Hydration: Drink cooling beverages (coconut water, buttermilk).
Avoid Overexertion: Too much heat can reduce sperm quality.
Diet: Sweet, juicy fruits and light meals.

Case Study: A young man experiencing low libido in summer found improvement after including rose petal jam and cooling herbs like Shatavari in his diet.

Monsoon (Varsha Ritu – September to October)
Immunity Boosters: Tulsi, honey, and Chyawanprash.
Light Diet: Avoid excessive dairy and fried foods.
Massage: Regular oil massage prevents Vata imbalance.

"वातः पित्तं कफश्चैव ऋतुविपर्ययेन तु।
स्वस्थस्य रक्षणं तस्माद्वतु अनुसरणं परम्॥"
(One must adapt to seasonal changes to maintain health.)

Autumn (Sharad Ritu – October to November)
Rejuvenation Therapy: Panchakarma & Rasayana therapy.

Herbs: Safed Musli & Brahmi enhance energy and mental clarity.
Diet: Ghee, dairy, and saffron-rich foods.
Winter (Hemanta & Shishira Ritu – December to February)
Strength Building: Heavier foods (urad dal, nuts, sesame seeds).
Warming Herbs: Ashwagandha, Gokshura, and Pippali.

Exercise: Intense strength training to channel energy.
Metaphor:
"Winter is like old age; proper nourishment keeps the fire burning."

Conclusion: Balance is the Key
Optimal sexual health is not about temporary fixes but a disciplined lifestyle. By following a structured daily routine (Dinacharya) and adapting to seasonal changes (Ritucharya), one can maintain vitality, balance hormones, and ensure a fulfilling intimate.

"As gold purified in fire shines more brightly, so does the disciplined life bring out the best in a person."

Chapter 24

AYURVEDIC DIET & NUTRITIONAL FOR SEXUAL HEALTH

Sexual energy is a direct reflection of overall health. Ayurveda considers it the essence of Shukra Dhatu, the final and most refined tissue in the body, responsible for vitality, fertility, and stamina. Modern nutritional science also recognizes the role of specific nutrients in boosting libido and reproductive health.

Quote:
"The food you eat can be either the safest and most powerful form of medicine or the slowest form of poison." – Ann Wigmore
Just as a river's flow determines the fertility of the land, our diet shapes our reproductive health. The right foods nourish sexual energy, while the wrong ones deplete it.

1. Ayurvedic Perspective

Nourishing the Shukra Dhatu In Ayurveda, reproductive energy is cultivated through a well-balanced diet that nourishes all bodily tissues. The concept of Vajikarana (aphrodisiac nutrition) is central to this.

"आहारसंभवं वस्तु रोगसंभवमथाह।"
(As food is, so is health; as improper diet is, so are diseases.)
Essential Ayurvedic Foods for Sexual Energy
Rasayana (Rejuvenating) Herbs & Foods
Ayurveda recommends powerful herbs that naturally enhance libido and stamina:
Ashwagandha reduces stress and enhances testosterone production.
Shatavari balances hormones and improves fertility.
Kaunch Beej (Mucuna Pruriens) increases dopamine and stamina.

Gokshura (Tribulus Terrestris) boosts testosterone and sexual performance.
Safed Musli is a natural aphrodisiac that increases sperm count.

Metaphor: "A well-oiled lamp gives a bright flame; similarly, a well-nourished body exhibits strong vitality."

Aphrodisiac Fruits & Nuts (Vajikarana Ahara)

Certain foods act as natural enhancers of sexual energy:
Dates and figs are rich in antioxidants that boost endurance.
Almonds and walnuts provide essential fatty acids for hormone production.

Pomegranate enhances blood flow to reproductive organs.

Case Study: A 35-year-old man suffering from low libido and stress-induced erectile dysfunction followed a diet rich in Ashwagandha, almonds, and saffron-infused milk. After three months, his testosterone levels improved by 20%, and his anxiety levels decreased significantly.

Dairy & Ghee for Ojas (Vital Energy)

According to Ayurveda, dairy is essential for reproductive health. Cow's milk is rich in calcium and zinc, while desi ghee lubricates internal tissues and enhances libido.

"दुग्धहितं श्रेष्ठं मेध्या बलवर्धनम् ॥"
(Milk is supreme; it enhances intellect and strength.)

Ayurvedic Spices for Libido
Saffron (Kesar) enhances mood and sexual performance.
Nutmeg (Jaiphal) acts as a natural aphrodisiac.
Cardamom (Elaichi) stimulates blood circulation, aiding stamina.

2. **Modern Nutritional Science**

Essential Nutrients for Sexual Health
Modern research supports the Ayurvedic principles, emphasizing the role of specific nutrients in enhancing reproductive function.
Key Nutrients & Their Benefits
Zinc (The Fertility Mineral)
Pumpkin seeds, sesame seeds, and oysters are rich sources of zinc, which boosts testosterone and sperm production. Studies confirm that zinc deficiency is linked to low libido and infertility.

Magnesium (Stress-Reliever for Better Performance)
Spinach, dark chocolate, and nuts are excellent sources of magnesium, which reduces cortisol (stress hormone) and improves blood circulation.

Omega-3 Fatty Acids (For Blood Flow & Hormone Balance)
Flaxseeds, walnuts, and salmon provide Omega-3s, which enhance dopamine levels and improve erectile function.

Metaphor: "A river must flow freely to sustain life; similarly, proper blood circulation is essential for reproductive health."
L-Arginine (A Natural Viagra)
Watermelon, peanuts, and lentils contain L-Arginine, an amino acid that expands blood vessels and enhances sexual performance.

Antioxidants (Protecting Sperm & Eggs from Damage)
Blueberries, green tea, and dark chocolate are rich in antioxidants that prevent oxidative stress, improving fertility.

Case Study: A couple struggling with infertility adopted a Mediterranean diet rich in antioxidants, Omega-3s, and zinc. Within six months, they noticed significant improvement in sperm motility and egg quality, leading to a successful conception.

3. **Ayurvedic & Modern Nutrition**

A Perfect Blend A holistic approach to sexual health integrates both Ayurvedic and modern dietary principles.
Morning Routine: Start the day with saffron-infused milk, soaked almonds, and dates.
Breakfast: Consume ghee-roasted oats with honey and banana for sustained energy.
Lunch: Include dal, ghee, and seasonal vegetables along with zinc-rich pumpkin seeds.
Evening Boost: Drink herbal tea with Ashwagandha and enjoy a small piece of dark chocolate for antioxidants.
Dinner: Opt for light khichdi with cumin and coriander, paired with a protein-rich source like salmon or tofu.

Conclusion: Balance is the Key to Vitality
Sexual energy is not just about short-term performance, but long-term nourishment through the right foods, herbs, and lifestyle. By integrating Ayurvedic wisdom with modern nutritional science, one can ensure a lifetime of vigor, passion, and well-being.

Chapter 25

SEXUAL DETOX & PANCHAKARMA THERAPY

Sexual energy is one of the most powerful life forces. However, in the modern world, it is often depleted due to stress, unhealthy diet, excessive indulgence, and mental toxicity. Ayurveda emphasizes that periodic detoxification is essential to restore vitality, purify reproductive tissues, and rejuvenate Shukra Dhatu (the reproductive essence).

Panchakarma, the supreme detox therapy of Ayurveda, plays a vital role in eliminating accumulated toxins (Ama) and restoring balance in the body and mind.

Quote:
"Your body is a temple, but only if you treat It as one." — Astrid Alauda
Just as a river becomes polluted over time and needs cleansing to flow freely, our sexual energy can be blocked by toxins and impurities, requiring periodic detoxification.

1. The Need for Sexual Detox in Modern Life

Modern lifestyle habits—processed food, alcohol, excessive digital exposure, stress, and lack of proper sleep—lead to the accumulation of toxins. This results in:
Low libido and sexual fatigue
Hormonal imbalances
Infertility and erectile dysfunction
Mental and emotional exhaustion

Blocked Nadis (energy channels), restricting the free flow of Prana l
"शुद्धशरीरस्य निरोगता"

(A cleansed body is free from diseases.)
Periodic detoxification allows Shukra Dhatu to regenerate, restoring passion, stamina, and overall well-being.

Case Study: A 40-year-old corporate professional experiencing chronic fatigue, low libido, and mental exhaustion underwent Panchakarma therapy at an Ayurvedic center. After completing Virechana (therapeutic purgation) and Basti (medicated enema), his energy levels improved, and he reported enhanced libido and mental clarity within a few weeks.

2. **Panchakarma**: The Ultimate Sexual Detox

Panchakarma consists of five purification procedures that deeply cleanse the body and mind. These therapies help eliminate Ama (toxins), balance Doshas, and restore Ojas (vital energy).

"शुद्धे हि धातुषु नरः सुखमेधते।"

(When body tissues are pure, one experiences happiness and vitality.)
The Five Panchakarma Therapies for Sexual Detox

a. **Vamana (Therapeutic Emesis)** – Removing Excess Kapha
Clears excess mucus and toxins, enhancing testosterone production and mental clarity.
Best for individuals with low libido due to lethargy and obesity.

B. **Virechana (Therapeutic Purgation)** – Purging Pitta Toxins
Eliminates toxins from the liver and intestines, which is crucial for hormonal balance and semen quality.
Ideal for those suffering from inflammation, erectile dysfunction, and skin issues.

Metaphor: "Just as a clogged drain needs a deep cleanse to function properly, Virechana purifies the body's metabolic pathways for optimal vitality."

C. **Basti (Medicated Enema)** – The King of Detox
Strengthens reproductive organs and nervous system.
Used for treating premature ejaculation, low sperm count, and weak libido.
Helps in mental detoxification, improving focus and emotional stability.

Case Study: A 33-year-old man with stress-induced sexual dysfunction underwent a 30-day Basti therapy. Post-treatment, he reported better erection quality, increased stamina, and improved mental focus.

D. **Nasya (Nasal Therapy)** – Clearing Mental Toxins
Clears mental fatigue, anxiety, and emotional stress that hinder sexual performance.
Medicated oils like Brahmi and Shatavari Nasya are used to sharpen the mind and balance hormones.

E. **Raktamokshana (Bloodletting)** – Purifying the Circulatory System
Enhances blood circulation, ensuring proper oxygenation of reproductive organs.
Useful for conditions like varicocele and toxin-induced erectile dysfunction.

3. Ayurvedic Lifestyle & Sexual Detox

To maintain post-Panchakarma benefits, Ayurveda recommends a Sattvic (pure) diet and disciplined lifestyle.
Daily Detox Practices for Sexual Energy

Warm Water & Lemon – Flushes out toxins and enhances metabolism.
Ashwagandha & Shatavari Milk – Restores Ojas and Shukra Dhatu.
Oil Pulling & Nasya Therapy – Clears mental fog and improves focus.

Sun Salutation (Surya Namaskar) – Improves blood flow and flexibility.
Abhyanga (Self-Massage with Herbal Oils) – Nourishes the nervous system and improves sexual vitality.
Pranayama & Meditation – Clears emotional blockages, reducing stress-related sexual disorders.

"युक्ताहारविहारस्य युक्तचेष्टस्य कर्मसु।"
(A balanced diet and lifestyle lead to longevity and vitality.) – Bhagavad Gita

4. Foods & Herbs to Support Sexual Detox

After undergoing Panchakarma, consuming detoxifying and rejuvenating foods is essential for sustained sexual energy.

Detoxifying Foods
Triphala – Cleanses intestines and improves digestion.
Neem & Tulsi – Purifies blood and enhances immunity.
Amla (Indian Gooseberry) – Rejuvenates reproductive tissues.
Ginger & Turmeric – Reduce inflammation and improve circulation.
Rejuvenating Herbs (Rasayana)
Shilajit – Restores lost vigor and testosterone levels.
Safed Musli – Acts as a natural aphrodisiac.
Kaunch Beej – Enhances sperm quality and motility.
Bala & Gokshura – Strengthen reproductive organs.

Metaphor: "A fertile land produces healthy crops; similarly, a cleansed and nourished body ensures peak reproductive health."

5. The Mental & Emotional Detox for Sexual Well-being

Sexual energy is not just physical; it is deeply connected to the mind and emotions. Emotional toxicity from stress, guilt, or trauma can hinder natural sexual functions.

Practices for Mental Detox:
Chanting "Om Namah Shivaya" – Harmonizes energy and calms the mind.
Journaling & Self-Reflection – Releases emotional baggage.
Gratitude Practice – Shifts focus from stress to positivity.
Celibacy (Brahmacharya) Detox – Periodic abstinence recharges sexual energy and enhances mental clarity.

Conclusion: A Path to Purity & Vitality
Sexual detox is not just about cleansing the body but realigning with nature's rhythm. By integrating Panchakarma, a sattvic diet, and mental detox practices, one can experience heightened sexual energy, mental clarity, and emotional balance.

Chapter 26

STRESS, ANXIETY & THEIR IMPACT ON SEXUALITY

Intimacy is the foundation of human relationships, yet it is fragile. In today's fast-paced world, stress and anxiety have become major disruptors of emotional and physical connection. Ayurveda and modern psychology agree that mental distress directly impacts sexual desire, performance, and overall well-being.

Quote:
"The greatest weapon against stress is our ability to choose one thought over another." – William James
Just as a flame needs a calm breeze to burn steadily, intimacy needs a peaceful mind to flourish. Stress and anxiety act as storms that extinguish the warmth of passion and connection.

1.   How Stress & Anxiety Affect Intimacy

Modern research and ancient wisdom both confirm that psychological distress leads to physiological dysfunctions. Chronic stress causes:
Cortisol Overload – Suppresses testosterone and estrogen, reducing libido.
Nervous System Imbalance – Activates the fight-or-flight response, diverting energy away from intimacy.
Emotional Disconnection – Increases irritability, reducing emotional bonding.
Performance Anxiety – Triggers erectile dysfunction and premature ejaculation.

"मन एव मनुष्याणां कारणं बन्धमोक्षयोः।"
(The mind alone is responsible for both bondage and liberation.) –

Yoga Vasistha
When the mind is stressed, intimacy suffers; when it is calm, love and passion thrive.

2. The Science behind Stress & Sexual Dysfunction

A. The Role of Cortisol: The Libido Killer

Chronic stress raises cortisol levels, disrupting the balance of reproductive hormones.
Elevated cortisol lowers testosterone in men and estrogen in women, leading to a decrease in libido.
Excess cortisol also leads to fatigue, weight gain, and mood swings, further diminishing sexual desire.

B. The Nervous System & The Fight-or-Flight Response

When the brain perceives stress, it prioritizes survival over reproduction.
Blood flow is diverted from the reproductive organs to the muscles, affecting arousal and performance.
Over time, this leads to erectile dysfunction, vaginal dryness, and delayed orgasm.

Case Study: A 35-year-old entrepreneur experiencing performance anxiety and erectile dysfunction sought Ayurvedic therapy. Through meditation, Ashwagandha supplementation, and Panchakarma detox, he regained confidence and reported restored libido and stronger emotional connection with his partner.

3. Anxiety: The Silent Killer of Intimacy

Anxiety is the constant anticipation of failure, rejection, or embarrassment, which destroys the spontaneity and joy of intimacy.

Effects of Anxiety on Sexual Health:

Negative Thought Cycles – Fear of failure leads to self-doubt, affecting performance.
Overthinking & Guilt – Cultural conditioning and past experiences create emotional baggage.
Hormonal Imbalance – Anxiety increases adrenaline, which reduces arousal.
Disconnection from Partner – Creates communication barriers, making emotional bonding difficult.

"चिन्ता जायते दुःखं, नाशयते सुखं नरं।"
(Anxiety gives rise to sorrow and destroys happiness.)

Metaphor: "A river flows freely when unobstructed. But when blocked by stones of fear and doubt, its flow weakens—just like intimacy hindered by anxiety."

3. Healing Intimacy Through Ayurvedic & Psychological Practices

A. Balancing the Mind Through Ayurveda

1. Medhya Rasayanas (Brain Tonic Herbs) for Stress Relief
Brahmi & Shankhpushpi – Enhance cognitive function and reduce stress.
Ashwagandha & Tagara – Reduce cortisol, improving libido and stamina.
Shatavari – Regulates hormones and supports emotional stability.

Case Study: A 28-year-old woman suffering from low libido due to anxiety was given Shatavari and Brahmi Rasayana. Within a month, her stress levels decreased, and she reported enhanced intimacy and confidence.

2. Abhyanga (Ayurvedic Oil Massage) to Soothe the Nervous System

Sesame oil massage nourishes the nerves and reduces anxiety.
Shirodhara (oil pouring on the forehead) activates the parasympathetic system, promoting relaxation.

3. Panchakarma Detox for Emotional Healing

Nasya therapy (nasal oil drops) clears mental fog and stress.
Basti (medicated enema) removes toxins affecting the reproductive system.

B. Psychological Practices for Enhancing Intimacy

1. Mindfulness & Breathwork

Diaphragmatic Breathing (Pranayama) — Activates the parasympathetic nervous system, reducing stress.
Anulom Vilom & Bhramari Pranayama — Improve oxygen flow to the brain, enhancing emotional balance.

2. Emotional Detox Through Communication

Open discussions about desires, fears, and expectations create a safe emotional space.
Active listening fosters trust and connection.

"स्नेहाद्विना न जीवनं, न च सुखस्य कारणं।"

(Without affection, life lacks meaning, and happiness remains elusive.)

3.   Tantra & Yogic Techniques for Deeper Connection

Yoga postures like Bhujangasana, Vajrasana, and Padmasana activate the root chakra, boosting sexual energy.
Tantric Gazing — Looking into a partner's eyes without words enhances emotional intimacy.

Metaphor: "A musical instrument must be tuned before it can create harmony. Similarly, a mind free of stress creates the melody of true intimacy."

5. The Role of Diet in Stress-Free Intimacy

Foods That Reduce Stress & Enhance Intimacy
Almonds & Walnuts — Boost serotonin, improving mood.
Dark Chocolate — Reduces cortisol, enhancing libido.
Bananas & Avocados — Provide B vitamins essential for dopamine production.
Warm Saffron & Ashwagandha Milk — Enhances relaxation and stamina.

Foods to Avoid

Caffeine & Alcohol — Increase anxiety and hormonal imbalance.
Processed Sugars — Disrupt serotonin levels, causing mood swings.
Shloka on Balanced Diet:
"युक्ताहारविहारस्य युक्तचेष्टस्य कर्मसु।"
(Balanced diet and lifestyle lead to vitality and longevity.) — Bhagavad Gita

Conclusion: The Path to Stress-Free Intimacy

Stress and anxiety are intimacy killers, but they are not invincible. Through Ayurvedic wisdom, psychological resilience, and conscious living, one can restore passion, connection, and confidence in intimacy.

Chapter 27

HOW PORN & SCREEN TIME AFFECT INTIMACY

The digital age has brought immense advancements, but it has also introduced new challenges to intimacy and sexual health. The overuse of screens and pornography is reshaping human relationships, leading to sexual dysfunction, emotional disconnect, and psychological distress.

Quote:
"Technology is a useful servant but a dangerous master." — Christian Lous Lange

Just as fire can be a source of warmth or destruction, digital consumption can either enhance or ruin relationships. When overindulged, it creates a disconnect between real intimacy and artificial stimulation.

1. The Impact of Pornography on Sexual Health

A. Rewiring the Brain: The Dopamine Trap
Pornography triggers artificial surges of dopamine, the brain's pleasure chemical.

Over time, the brain becomes desensitized, needing stronger, more extreme content to feel aroused.

This leads to low libido, erectile dysfunction (ED), and unrealistic expectations in real relationships.

"न हि कश्चित् क्षणमपि जातु तिष्ठत्यकर्मकृत्।"
(The mind cannot remain inactive even for a moment; it follows what it is trained to seek.) — Bhagavad Gita 3.5

If one constantly feeds the mind digital fantasies, real intimacy starts feeling dull and unsatisfying.

Case Study: A 27-year-old male suffering from porn-induced erectile dysfunction (PIED) was unable to feel arousal with his real partner despite being physically healthy. Through Brahmacharya practices, dopamine detox, and Ayurvedic Rasayanas, he regained normal sexual function within four months.

2. Screen Time & Its Effect on Sexual Energy

A. Blue Light Disrupts Hormonal Balance

Excessive screen exposure before bedtime reduces melatonin, affecting sleep and testosterone production.
Poor sleep lowers libido and leads to fatigue, irritability, and sexual dysfunction.

B. Emotional Disconnect Due to Digital Overload

Constant scrolling reduces face-to-face emotional bonding.
Social media creates unrealistic comparisons, leading to dissatisfaction in relationships.
Partners feel ignored, leading to resentment and reduced intimacy.

"योगश्चित्तवृत्ति निरोध: ।"
(Yoga is the control of mental distractions.) – Patanjali Yoga Sutra 1.2
When attention is scattered between multiple digital distractions, true intimacy weakens.

Metaphor: "A candle cannot burn brightly in strong wind. Likewise, love and passion cannot thrive when constantly disturbed by digital distractions."

3. How Porn Addiction Leads to Sexual Dysfunction

A. The Cycle of Porn-Induced Erectile Dysfunction (PIED)

Excessive porn consumption overstimulates the brain.
Real intimacy feels less exciting compared to virtual fantasies.
The body develops "arousal dependency" on digital content.
Erectile dysfunction, low libido, and delayed ejaculation occur in real encounters.

Case Study: A 35-year-old IT professional, addicted to pornography since his teens, experienced severe intimacy issues. Through digital detox, Vajikarana herbs like Ashwagandha, and Brahmacharya meditation, he revived his relationship within six months.

Shloka on Restraining Desires:
"वशे हि यस्येन्द्रियाणि तस्य प्रज्ञा प्रतिष्ठिता।"
(He who has control over his senses possesses true wisdom.) – Bhagavad Gita 2.61
By controlling sensory indulgence, one can regain lost vigor and deep intimacy.

4. Ayurvedic Solutions to Reclaim Sexual Health

A. Vajikarana Rasayanas (Aphrodisiac Herbs)

Ashwagandha – Lowers stress, boosts testosterone.
Shatavari – Enhances libido and emotional bonding.
Kaunch Beej (Mucuna Pruriens) – Increases dopamine naturally.
Gokshura (Tribulus Terrestris) – Improves circulation to reproductive organs.

B. Detoxing the Brain from Pornography

Dopamine Fasting – A 30-day break from digital stimulation resets the brain.
Meditation & Pranayama – Helps regain focus and emotional stability.
Abhyanga (Oil Massage) – Nourishes the nervous system, reducing anxiety.

"तस्मात् त्वमिन्द्रियाण्यादौ नियम्य भरतर्षभ।"
(Therefore, O Arjuna, control the senses first to attain true mastery.) – Bhagavad Gita 3.41
When desires are regulated, natural intimacy and confidence return.

5. Rebuilding Real Intimacy in the Digital Age

A. Practical Steps for Digital Detox in Relationships
No Screens in the Bedroom – Keep phones out of intimate spaces.
Daily "Eye Contact Ritual" – Spend 5 minutes looking into your partner's eyes without distractions.
Tech-Free Evenings – At least 2 hours before bed, switch off screens.
Engage in Physical Activities Together – Yoga, walking, or dancing increases bonding.

B. The Power of Slow Love

Digital consumption promotes instant gratification, while true intimacy requires patience and deep connection.
Tantra practices like synchronized breathing and mindful touch restore lost passion.

"सौहार्दं सर्वभूतानां यस्तु कुर्वीत स योगी।"
(One who cultivates harmony in all relationships is a true Yogi.)

Conclusion: The Path to Conscious Intimacy

In the digital age, intimacy is being replaced by instant stimulation. By understanding the impact of excessive screen time and pornography, one can reclaim natural sexual health and deeper relationships.

Chapter 28

THE ART OF EMOTIONAL & SPIRITUAL CONNECTION

In a world increasingly focused on physical gratification, the concept of Sacred Sexuality offers a return to the soulful union of body, mind, and spirit. It transcends lust and enters a space where two individuals connect emotionally, spiritually, and energetically — leading not only to pleasure, but also to inner healing, transformation, and higher consciousness.

Quote: "Sexual energy is the creative energy of the universe. It can destroy or awaken the divine within." – Osho

Just as fire can burn or illuminate, sexuality can either consume or elevate when directed with awareness.

1. Understanding Sacred Sexuality

Sacred sexuality is not just about sex — it is about the integration of love, respect, and soul-level connection. It's where intimacy becomes a spiritual practice, a sacred dance between two energies.

"यत्र नार्यस्तु पूज्यन्ते रमन्ते तत्र देवता: ।"
(Where women are honored, divinity blossoms there.) — Manusmriti 3.56
Sacred sexuality honors both the masculine and the feminine, as equal partners in divine union — not as objects, but as sacred reflections of the divine.

2. Emotional Connection: The Gateway to Sacred Union

A fulfilling sexual experience begins emotionally. When partners are emotionally safe, loved, and seen — their bodies respond naturally and deeply.

Case Study: A couple in their 40s, on the verge of separation, began practicing daily emotional check-ins and eye-gazing meditations. Over time, their emotional intimacy rekindled, leading to a restoration of sexual harmony and spiritual closeness.

Metaphor: "Trying to ignite sexual fire without emotional fuel is like lighting a lamp with no oil."

Quote: "To touch the soul of another human being is to walk on holy ground." – Stephen Covey

3. Spiritual Connection: The Role of Energy & Tantra
In many spiritual traditions — especially Tantra and Ayurveda — sexual energy is revered as Shakti, the powerful life-force. When shared consciously, it awakens the Kundalini energy, which travels through the chakras and opens the heart and consciousness.

"कुण्डलिनी शक्तिस्तु सूक्ष्मरूपेण संस्थिता।"
(Kundalini Shakti lies dormant at the base, awaiting awakening to ascend toward divinity.)
Sacred sex becomes a form of worship, where the partner is not just a body, but a temple of divine energy.

Practice: Tantric Breathing: Breathing in sync while holding gaze.
Yab-Yum Posture: Seated connection of divine masculine and feminine.
Heart-to-Heart Touch: Slow, mindful physical contact with spiritual awareness.

4. The Role of Mindfulness in Sacred Sexuality

Presence is the essence of sacred connection. When partners are fully in the moment — with no expectations, no judgments — time dissolves, and so do the ego barriers.

Metaphor: "Sacred sex is like a raga played on a sitar — slow, rhythmic, and rich in soul. It is not noise, it is music."
"सर्वं खल्विदं ब्रह्म।"
(All this — the seen and unseen — is divine.) – Chandogya Upanishad 3.14.1

Even the body, its desires, and its union — are part of the divine experience when approached with reverence.

5. Ayurvedic View: Balancing Doshas for Deep Connection

In Ayurveda, sexual energy (Shukra Dhatu) is the essence of all tissues. A sacred union requires balanced Vata (communication), Pitta (passion), and Kapha (emotional bonding).

Rituals for Sacred Union:
Abhyanga (Oil Massage) before intimacy to balance Vata and build connection
Aphrodisiac herbs like Shatavari (for women) and Ashwagandha (for men) to enhance vitality and calm the mind
Nasya or Shirodhara for calming the nervous system and promoting emotional openness

6. Sacred Celibacy vs. Sacred Sexuality

In sacred traditions, celibacy and sacred sexuality are not opposites, but two sides of the same coin. One is the retention and redirection of energy inward, the other is the conscious exchange of energy outward.

Quote from the Kama Sutra:
"Pleasure should be with awareness, not with indulgence. In pleasure lies both liberation and bondage."
Metaphor: "Sex is a sword — in an undisciplined hand it wounds, but in the hands of a master it becomes an instrument of honor."

7. Healing Through Sacred Sexuality

Sacred sex is not only pleasurable, but also deeply healing. When trauma, shame, or past wounds are gently held in the sacred presence of a loving partner, they begin to dissolve.

Case Study: A woman with a history of sexual trauma reported emotional release and spiritual awakening after months of guided Tantric practice, which included breathwork, bodywork, and mantra chanting with her partner.

Conclusion: Sacred Union is a Journey, Not a Destination
Sacred sexuality is a devotional path, not a performance. It is about awareness, reverence, connection, and surrender. It restores wholeness, heals emotional wounds, and leads to spiritual expansion.

SECTION 6

INTEGRATING MODERN SCIENCE & AYURVEDA

Chapter 29

HORMONE THERAPY VS AYURVEDIC RASAYANAS

The modern world faces increasing health challenges like hormonal imbalances, infertility, aging, and stress. In this context, two approaches have gained prominence: Hormone Therapy from modern medicine and Rasayana Therapy from Ayurveda. While hormone therapy offers rapid relief, Ayurvedic rasayanas focus on long-term rejuvenation.

1. Philosophy and Principle

Hormone Therapy (Modern Medicine)

Mechanism: Direct supplementation or manipulation of hormones (e.g., estrogen, testosterone, insulin).
Philosophy: Treat the symptoms by replacing or altering the deficient hormones.
Metaphor: Hormone therapy is like a crutch for a limping leg—it supports but does not strengthen.

Ayurvedic Rasayanas

Mechanism: Rejuvenating herbs and lifestyle practices to restore internal balance and promote ojas (vitality).
Philosophy: Heal the root cause by balancing doshas and enhancing the dhatus (tissues).
A refined and well-structured Sanskrit version of your verse is:

"रसायनं च तत् ज्ञेयं यद् बलवर्धनं परम्।
आयुः सत्त्वबलोपेतं रसायनं तत् स्मृतम्
Charaka Samhita

(That which enhances longevity, intelligence, strength and vitality is called Rasayana.)

Metaphor: Rasayana is like nurturing the soil so that the plant flourishes naturally.

2. Ingredients & Substances

Hormone Therapy:
Uses synthetic or bioidentical hormones (e.g., HRT, insulin, thyroid hormones).
Potential for side effects like cancer risk, cardiovascular issues, dependency.

Rasayanas

Herbal and mineral compounds like Ashwagandha, Shatavari, Brahmi, Amalaki.
Promote natural hormone regulation without synthetic introduction.

Case Study – PCOS Patient: A 28-year-old woman with PCOS was on birth control pills and metformin. Side effects included weight gain and mood swings. Switched to Ayurvedic treatment with Shatavari, Triphala, and Panchakarma therapy. Within 6 months, hormonal levels normalized and menstrual cycle became regular. Outcome: Sustainable recovery without side effects.

3. Side Effects vs. Side Benefits

Hormone Therapy

Side Effects: Blood clots, mood disorders, increased cancer risk.
Needs regular monitoring and adjustment.

Quote: "Every silver bullet comes with a cost in medicine. Hormones are no exception." — Dr. Andrew Weil

Rasayanas:

Side Benefits: Improved immunity, better digestion, enhanced memory.

Holistic healing of body, mind, and spirit.

"दीर्घमायुर् बलं मेधां स्मृतिमारोग्यमुत्तमम्।
प्रज्ञां च मे प्रयच्छन्तु रसायनानि सर्वदा॥"

Ashtanga Hridaya

(May the rasayanas bless me with long life, strength, intellect, memory, and perfect health.)

4. Long-Term Effects and Sustainability

Hormone Therapy

Quick fixes but may cause dependency.
Often treats the symptom rather than root cause.

Metaphor: Like painting over rust – the problem re-emerges.

Rasayanas

Rejuvenate body systems gradually.
Promote long-term health and resilience.

Metaphor: Like rainwater seeping into roots—slow, steady, and life-giving.

5. Personalization and Preventive Potential

Hormone Therapy:
Based on lab tests and standardized dosing.
Limited personalization; focuses on cure.

Rasayanas:
Tailored to individual prakriti (constitution), age, lifestyle, and season.
Strong focus on prevention (swasthasya swasthya rakshanam).
"यस्यान् रोगो न भवति, तं रोगिणं न वदन्ति ॥"
Sushruta Samhita
(One who does not fall sick is not called a patient.)

7. Integrative Potential

Many modern integrative doctors now combine the two: using hormone therapy for acute conditions and rasayanas for sustainable healing.

Case Study – Menopausal Health:
A woman aged 52 used HRT for 2 years but experienced hot flashes and depression. An integrative physician introduced Ashwagandha, Yoga, and a Satvik diet. HRT was gradually reduced. Quality of life improved with more energy, calmness, and hormonal balance.

Conclusion

Hormone Therapy:
Fast and effective but potentially risky.
Best for acute or life-threatening imbalances.

Ayurvedic Rasayanas

Slow but deep-acting and safe.
Best for long-term health, prevention, and holistic rejuvenation.
 "Nature heals. Modern medicine intervenes. A wise healer knows when to use both." — Dr. Vasant Lad

Chapter 30

VIAGRA VS AYURVEDIC VAJIKARANA DRAVYAS

Sexual health is not just a physical concern—it's deeply tied to one's emotional, psychological, and spiritual well-being. In today's fast-paced world, solutions to sexual dysfunction often take the form of quick-fix pharmaceuticals like Viagra, while ancient Indian wisdom offers a holistic rejuvenation through Vajikarana, one of the eight major branches of Ayurveda.

This analysis explores the contrast between these two paradigms—one focused on temporary performance, the other on sustained vitality.

Two Philosophies of Healing

Viagra represents the modern scientific approach: identify the symptom, target the mechanism, and stimulate the response. It works by increasing blood flow through the inhibition of an enzyme (PDE5), resulting in a temporary erection. The purpose is performance-centric.

Metaphor: Viagra is like a firecracker—intense, short-lived, and explosive.

On the other hand, Vajikarana is rooted in the ancient Ayurvedic philosophy of nurturing the "Shukra Dhatu" (reproductive tissue), building "Ojas" (life energy), and restoring balance in the mind, body, and spirit. Its purpose is transformational and life-affirming. Shloka from Charaka Samhita:

"Vajikaranam cha tat jneyam, yenedam tarunam vapuḥ,
Prabhootam sukramayati, shaktam strishu pramoditum."

(That which restores youth, increases semen, and empowers joyful union is known as Vajikarana.)

Nature of Action: Immediate vs. Enduring

Viagra acts swiftly—usually within 30 to 60 minutes—producing an erection sufficient for intercourse. However, it does not address the root causes of sexual dysfunction, such as stress, hormonal imbalance, or lack of vitality. Its effects wear off within a few hours, and repeated use may lead to dependence or psychological pressure.

Metaphor: Viagra is like borrowing energy on credit—you may pay the interest in side effects.
In contrast, Vajikarana herbs like Ashwagandha, Safed Musli, Kapikacchu, and Shilajit work slowly but profoundly. Over weeks or months, they rebuild the body's core vitality, enhance testosterone naturally, calm the mind, and increase sexual confidence.

Metaphor: Vajikarana is like tilling a field and planting seeds—it takes time, but the harvest is rich and nourishing.

Beyond the Body: Emotional and Psychological Effects
Modern medicine often isolates sexual dysfunction from the rest of life. A man is treated for ED without attention to his diet, sleep, emotions, or relationships. Viagra becomes a performance enhancer—not a life enhancer.
Quote: "Modern medicine treats erection, not connection."

Ayurveda, however, regards sexuality as sacred. It advocates for purity of thought, healthy relationships, balanced diet, yoga, and discipline (Brahmacharya) for optimal sexual health.
Shloka from Sushruta Samhita:
"Brahmacharyam aharatwam, nidra nityam yathavidhi,

Shuddha achara manushyānām, vajikaranam ucyate."
(Celibacy in moderation, appropriate diet, proper sleep, and noble conduct—these are true aphrodisiacs.)

Case Studies and Real-Life Impact

Case 1 – The Executive's Escape:

A 40-year-old corporate professional suffering from ED and anxiety relied on Viagra, but began to feel emotionally disconnected and physically drained. Upon shifting to Vajikarana therapy—Ashwagandha, Brahmi, and Abhyanga (oil therapy)—his vitality returned within 2 months. Anxiety subsided, and he began experiencing natural arousal and deeper emotional intimacy.

Case 2 – Restoring Fertility Naturally:

A 36-year-old man with low sperm count (12 million/ml) opted for Ayurvedic therapy with Kaunch Beej, Shilajit, and Panchakarma (detox therapies). After 3 months, his count improved to 35 million/ml, along with marked improvement in energy and libido—without any pharmaceutical drugs.

Side Effects vs. Side Benefits

Viagra is known to cause headaches, nasal congestion, flushing, and sometimes visual disturbances. There is also the psychological side effect of performance pressure and the risk of becoming reliant on the pill.

Quote: "Sometimes the mind gets addicted before the body does." – Dr. Deepak Chopra

In contrast, Vajikarana offers side benefits: improved immunity, better sleep, enhanced clarity, youthful energy, and deeper connection with the partner.

Cultural Context and Social Acceptance

Viagra is often used in secrecy and viewed as a sign of weakness or aging. Vajikarana, however, has a cultural and spiritual legitimacy in India. It is not just accepted but revered—taught as an Upaveda (sub-Veda) and prescribed to kings, sages, and householders.

Conclusion: Two Roads to Intimacy
Viagra and Vajikarana both aim to address sexual dysfunction, but they differ in philosophy, action, and outcome. Viagra offers speed, stimulation, and symptom relief. Vajikarana offers depth, rejuvenation, and sustainable transformation.

 "Viagra awakens the body. Vajikarana awakens the soul." – Dr. Mukesh Aggarwal

Ultimately, the choice depends on whether one seeks a spark—or a lasting flame.

Chapter 31

AYURVEDA IN ADDRESSING SEXUAL DISORDERS

Sexual health is a cornerstone of overall well-being, yet modern lifestyles, stress, poor diet, and environmental toxins have led to an epidemic of sexual disorders—erectile dysfunction (ED), premature ejaculation (PE), low libido, and infertility. Conventional medicine often provides quick-fix solutions like Viagra, testosterone replacement, or antidepressants, but these do not address the root cause.

Ayurveda, the 5,000-year-old science of life, offers a more sustainable approach, focusing on rejuvenation, balance, and vitality through Vajikarana Chikitsa (aphrodisiac therapy). This article explores how Ayurveda can effectively address modern sexual disorders using herbs, diet, lifestyle modifications, detoxification therapies, and psychological healing.

Metaphor: Modern medicine is like painting over rust, while Ayurveda is like removing the rust and restoring the metal to its original shine.

Understanding Sexual Disorders from an Ayurvedic Perspective
In Ayurveda, sexual disorders are not isolated conditions but are linked to imbalances in the Tridoshas (Vata, Pitta, Kapha) and weakness in the Shukra Dhatu (reproductive tissue). Ayurveda recognizes:

Erectile Dysfunction (ED) – Caused by excess Vata (anxiety, overthinking, weakness) or Pitta (overexertion, excess heat).

Premature Ejaculation (PE) – A Vata disorder due to excessive nervous system activity.

Low Libido – A Kapha imbalance, often due to lethargy, obesity, or metabolic disorders.
Infertility – A complex issue linked to poor Shukra Dhatu, poor digestion (Agni), and emotional stress.

"वाजीकरण द्रव्याणि शुक्रं बलं च वर्धयेत्।
शुद्धं देहं मनो नित्यं, वयः स्थापन हेतवः॥"
Charaka Samhita (Chikitsa Sthana 2/1):
(Aphrodisiac herbs nourish the reproductive system, enhance strength, purify the body and mind, and maintain youthfulness.)

Ayurvedic Solutions to Sexual Disorders

1. Vajikarana Dravyas (Aphrodisiac Herbs & Foods)

Ayurveda prescribes natural remedies that nourish the body, calm the mind, and build lasting vigor:
Ashwagandha (Withania somnifera) – The ultimate rejuvenator, reduces stress-induced ED and improves sperm quality.
Shatavari (Asparagus racemosus) – Supports reproductive health in both men and women.
Kapikacchu (Mucuna pruriens) – Boosts dopamine, enhances sexual function, and treats premature ejaculation.
Safed Musli (Chlorophytum borivilianum) – Known as the "Indian Viagra," strengthens the reproductive system.
Shilajit (Purified Asphaltum) – Increases testosterone and stamina.

Case Study – The Entrepreneur's Revival:
A 38-year-old businessman faced stress-induced ED. He was prescribed Ashwagandha, Shatavari, and Kapikacchu, along with yoga and oil massage (Abhyanga). Within two months, his confidence, energy, and libido were naturally restored.

Metaphor: Ashwagandha is like the roots of a tree—it anchors you, giving you the strength to stand tall in life.

2. Panchakarma Therapy (Detox for Sexual Rejuvenation)

Toxins (Ama) accumulate in the body due to processed foods, alcohol, smoking, and pollution, leading to poor reproductive health. Panchakarma—Ayurveda's deep detox—removes these toxins and restores natural vitality.
Virechana (Purgation Therapy) – Clears Pitta toxins that affect sexual vigor.
Basti (Medicated Enema) – Balances Vata, treating PE and ED caused by stress.
Abhyanga (Oil Massage) – Reduces anxiety and enhances circulation to the reproductive organs.

"मलशुद्धिः जयेत् रोगान् सुखशुद्धं च वर्धयेत्।
देहस्य शोधनं नित्यं वृष्यं परम उच्यते॥"
Sushruta Samhita:
(Detoxification removes diseases, purifies pleasure, and enhances sexual vigor.)

3. Psychological Healing: The Mind-Body Connection

Sexual disorders are often psychogenic—caused by performance anxiety, stress, depression, or relationship issues. Ayurveda treats both the mind and body:
Brahmi & Gotu Kola – Calm the mind and reduce anxiety-related ED.
Yoga & Pranayama – Boost blood circulation and activate the parasympathetic nervous system, reducing stress-induced dysfunction.
Mantra & Meditation – Strengthen the subconscious mind to remove performance anxiety.

Case Study – The Young Husband's Struggle:
A 29-year-old newlywed suffered from performance anxiety-induced ED. After a regimen of Brahmi, yoga, and guided meditation, he developed confidence and restored his natural function within a month.

Quote from Dr. Deepak Chopra:
"True sexual health begins in the mind. When the mind is at ease, the body naturally follows."

4. Diet & Lifestyle: Nourishing Sexual Energy

A weak digestive fire (Agni) leads to poor absorption of nutrients, affecting sexual health. Ayurveda recommends:
Ghee, Almonds, and Sesame Seeds – Strengthen Shukra Dhatu.
Fruits like Dates, Figs, and Pomegranates – Enhance blood circulation to reproductive organs.
Avoid Excessive Spicy, Salty, and Oily Foods – These aggravate Pitta, leading to excess heat and sexual weakness.

"घृतं वृष्यं बल्यं च, नेत्र्यं मेध्यं परं मतम्।
रसायनं च रोगाणां, सर्वदोषहरं परम्॥"
Bhavaprakasha Nighantu
(Ghee is aphrodisiac, nourishing, improves intellect, and acts as a Rasayana (rejuvenator) for the entire body.)

Ayurveda vs. Modern Medicine: A Long-Term Solution

Modern medicine treats symptoms (e.g., Viagra for ED), while Ayurveda addresses the root cause by:
Restoring Shukra Dhatu
Strengthening the nervous system
Removing toxins (Ama)
Enhancing mind-body harmony

Metaphor: Viagra is like a shortcut through a jungle—it works for the moment but doesn't clear the path for future journeys. Ayurveda is like paving a road—it requires effort but lasts a lifetime.

Conclusion: A Return to Natural Virility
Ayurveda views sexual health as sacred, intertwined with physical, mental, and spiritual well-being. Instead of quick fixes, it offers a holistic path to true rejuvenation.
   "Sexual health is not about performance—it is about vitality, connection, and harmony." – Dr. Mukesh Aggarwal

By embracing Ayurveda's wisdom, one can reignite natural passion, restore youthful vigor, and cultivate a fulfilling, balanced life.

Chapter 32

INTEGRATIVE APPROACHES FOR A HEALTHY SEX LIFE

Sexual wellness is no longer limited to the treatment of dysfunctions; it is now seen as an essential part of physical, mental, and emotional well-being. The future of sexual health lies in integrative approaches that blend modern medicine, Ayurveda, psychology, nutrition, and lifestyle modifications.

As we move forward, the focus is shifting from mere performance enhancement to holistic well-being, stress management, emotional bonding, and longevity.

Metaphor: Sexual health is like a symphony—it requires harmony between the body, mind, and emotions to create a beautiful melody.

Understanding Sexual Wellness: A 360-Degree Approach

Sexual health is influenced by biological, psychological, social, and spiritual factors. Integrative wellness focuses on:

Physical Health – Hormonal balance, cardiovascular fitness, and reproductive health.

Mental Health – Stress reduction, emotional resilience, and relationship harmony.

Ayurvedic Wisdom – Strengthening Shukra Dhatu (reproductive tissue) and balancing the Tridoshas.

Modern Innovations – Biohacking, regenerative medicine, and natural supplements.

"वृष्याणि द्रव्याणि शुक्रं बलं च वर्धयेत्।
रसायनानि च नित्यं, वयः स्थापन हेतवः॥"
Charaka Samhita (Chikitsa Sthana 2.1):

(Aphrodisiac substances increase reproductive strength, act as rejuvenators, and support longevity.)

1. Ayurveda Meets Modern Medicine: The Best of Both Worlds
Modern Medical Advances in Sexual Wellness

Testosterone Optimization Therapy – Used for men with low testosterone.
Regenerative Medicine (Stem Cell & PRP Therapy) – Repairs tissues and enhances blood flow.
Neurotherapy & Cognitive Training – Improves sexual response and performance anxiety.
Biohacking & Supplements – L-arginine, zinc, and nitric oxide boosters enhance natural function.

Ayurvedic Solutions for Sexual Longevity

Ashwagandha – Reduces stress-induced erectile dysfunction (ED) and boosts testosterone.
Shatavari – Enhances libido and reproductive health in both men and women.
Shilajit – Known as the "Destroyer of Weakness," it enhances stamina and hormone balance.
Safed Musli – A natural Viagra that strengthens Shukra Dhatu.
Abhyanga (Oil Massage) & Panchakarma Detox – Rejuvenate the nervous system and reproductive organs.

Case Study – The CEO Who Regained His Passion:
A 42-year-old executive suffered from stress-induced ED. He combined Ashwagandha, Shilajit, and L-arginine supplements with breathwork and meditation. Within three months, he regained confidence and improved performance naturally.

Metaphor: Ayurveda is like a gardener who nourishes the soil for a long-lasting harvest, while modern medicine is like a sprinkler system that provides instant hydration.

3. The Psychology of Sexual Well-being

The Role of the Mind in Sexual Health
Stress, anxiety, and negative beliefs around sex are major contributors to dysfunction. The future of sexual wellness includes:
Mindfulness & Meditation – Enhances awareness and reduces performance anxiety.
Therapeutic Coaching – Sex therapy and cognitive-behavioral therapy (CBT) for psychological barriers.
Neuroscience & Emotional Intimacy – Strengthening dopamine and oxytocin levels to improve connection.
Quote by Dr. Deepak Chopra:
 "Sexual energy is the creative force of the universe; when balanced, it leads to vitality, connection, and joy."

Case Study – The Newlyweds' Transformation:
A 30-year-old couple faced relationship strain due to stress and lack of intimacy. With guided therapy, Ayurvedic aphrodisiacs, and mindfulness practices, their emotional and physical connection deepened.

4. Biohacking & Lifestyle Upgrades for Lifelong Sexual Vitality

The future of sexual wellness integrates science-backed biohacking strategies with traditional health practices:
Cold Therapy (Cryotherapy & Ice Baths) – Enhances testosterone and circulation.
Infrared Therapy & Red Light Therapy – Boosts nitric oxide and blood flow.

Intermittent Fasting & Ketogenic Diet – Reduces inflammation and improves hormone balance.
Superfoods for Sexual Energy – Maca root, ginseng, dark chocolate, and omega-3-rich foods.

Metaphor: Think of your body as a high-performance car—without the right fuel and maintenance, even the best engine will fail.

5.   Tantra & Conscious Sexuality: The Spiritual Dimension

Sexual health is not just physical—it has a spiritual aspect that Tantra and Eastern philosophies emphasize.
Tantric Practices for Deeper Intimacy
Pranayama & Breathwork – Expands pleasure and energy circulation.
Sacred Connection (Maithuna Yoga) – Transforms sex into a meditative experience.
Chakra Balancing – Activates the Swadhisthana (Sacral Chakra) for increased pasBhairav

"यत् सुखं ब्रह्म तत्तुल्यं, तत् सुखं स्वाध्याय जातम्॥"
Vijnana Bhairava Tantra:
(The bliss of divine consciousness is reflected in the bliss of sacred intimacy.)

Case Study – The Couple Who Reignited Passion:
A middle-aged couple struggling with fading intimacy embraced Tantric breathwork and Ayurvedic Vajikarana therapy. Their bond deepened beyond the physical, bringing emotional and spiritual fulfillment.

6. The Future of Sexual Wellness: A Paradigm Shift

The future of sexual health will be defined by:

Personalized Sexual Health Plans – Genetic and Ayurvedic-based recommendations.
AI & Wearable Tech – Devices monitoring hormone levels and stress responses.
Holistic Sexual Education – Schools and workplaces integrating sex-positive wellness programs.

Mainstream Integration of Ayurveda & Tantra – Acceptance of ancient wisdom in medical practices.

Metaphor: The future of sexual wellness is like an ecosystem—it thrives when physical, emotional, and spiritual elements work in balance.

Conclusion: A New Era of Sexual Well-being
Sexual health is not just about function—it is about connection, vitality, and holistic well-being. By embracing integrative solutions, we can cultivate lifelong passion, energy, and emotional fulfillment.

"Sexual wellness is not just an act; it is an art—an expression of balance, vitality, and love." – Dr. Mukesh Aggarwal